Preventing Sexual Diseases

ISSUES

Volume 96

Editor

Craig Donnellan

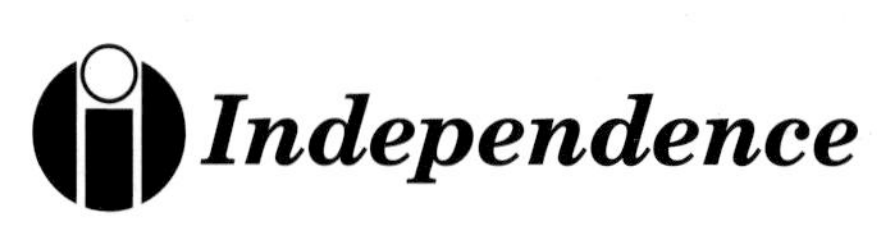

Educational Publishers
Cambridge

First published by Independence
PO Box 295
Cambridge CB1 3XP
England

British Library Cataloguing in Publication Data
Preventing Sexual Diseases – (Issues Series)
I. Donnellan, Craig II. Series
616.9'51

ISBN 1 86168 304 9

Printed in Great Britain
MWL Print Group Ltd

Typeset by
Claire Boyd

Cover
The illustration on the front cover is by
Pumpkin House.

CONTENTS

Chapter One: Sexual Health

Chapter Two: HIV & AIDS

Introduction

Preventing Sexual Diseases is the ninety-sixth volume in the ***Issues*** series. The aim of this series is to offer up-to-date information about important issues in our world.

Preventing Sexual Diseases looks at sexually transmitted diseases and sexual health.

The information comes from a wide variety of sources and includes:
Government reports and statistics
Newspaper reports and features
Magazine articles and surveys
Website material
Literature from lobby groups
and charitable organisations.

It is hoped that, as you read about the many aspects of the issues explored in this book, you will critically evaluate the information presented. It is important that you decide whether you are being presented with facts or opinions. Does the writer give a biased or an unbiased report? If an opinion is being expressed, do you agree with the writer?

Preventing Sexual Diseases offers a useful starting-point for those who need convenient access to information about the many issues involved. However, it is only a starting-point. At the back of the book is a list of organisations which you may want to contact for further information.

*****

Sexually transmitted infections

The facts

First things first

Sexually transmitted infections (STIs) are a major cause of ill health. They can also cause ectopic pregnancy (where an egg is fertilised and becomes implanted in the fallopian tube), and may also lead to infertility in both men and women.

Since 1995 there have been large increases in the number of people diagnosed with STIs, particularly women in their late teens and men in their early twenties. This may be because people are more aware of STIs and are visiting clinics to be tested.

What are the symptoms?

Symptoms vary between STIs and some have no symptoms at all. Where there are symptoms, these may include unusual discharge from the vagina or penis, heavy periods or bleeding between periods, pain or burning sensation when passing urine, rashes, itching or tingling around the genitals or anus.

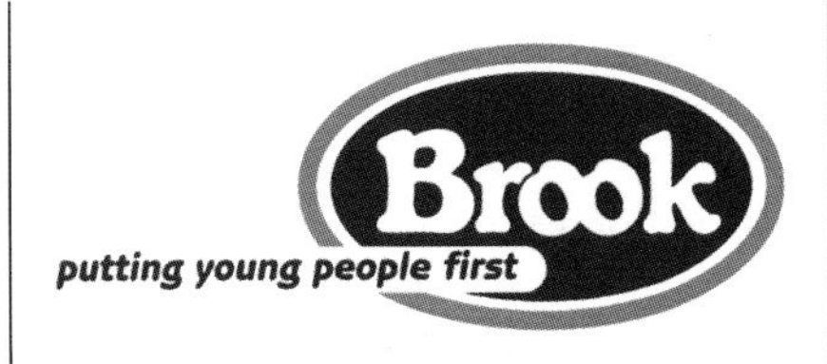

Tests and treatment

Most STIs can be easily diagnosed and treated at Genito-Urinary Medicine (GUM) clinics which are usually based in local hospitals. If you think you may have an STI, you can refer yourself to any GUM clinic for advice and treatment. The service is completely confidential and you don't have to go to your nearest clinic if you don't want to.

Contact our Ask Brook service to find a GUM clinic. Or look in the phone book under GUM or sexual health.

Tests for STIs vary. Some involve taking swabs from the cervix or tip of the penis. Others involve taking a blood sample.

Before being tested it is usual to see a health adviser who will discuss safer sex with you so that you can avoid infections in the future. Counselling is usually offered before testing for HIV so that you are prepared for the implications of the test result if it is positive.

If you test positive for any STI, the clinic will encourage you to talk to your current partner and, where relevant, previous partners, so that they can also be tested. If you prefer, the clinic can do this for you without revealing your identity. Most STIs are treatable with antibiotics.

Avoiding STIs

STIs are usually passed on by sex with an infected person though some can be passed on in other ways as well. They can be caught during oral, vaginal or anal sex.

Using a male or female condom every time you have sex will stop the transmission of most STIs. Condoms can be used in addition to another

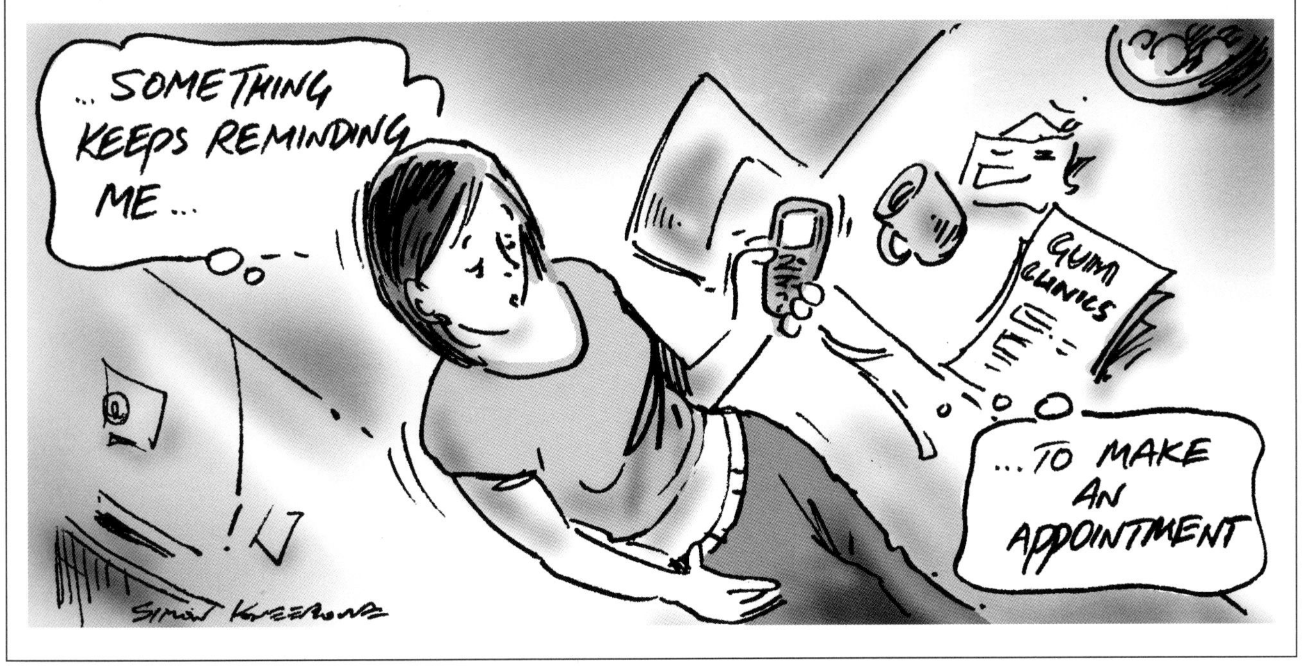

method of contraception, such as the pill, which does not protect against infections. This is often referred to as the 'double dutch' method.

Dental dams (small squares of latex) can also be used as a barrier during sex involving contact between the mouth and the vagina, or the mouth and the anus.

Condoms are easily available from Brook Centres (for under 25s) and family planning clinics, and dental dams are available from GUM clinics.

Types of STI

There are 25 types of sexually transmitted infection. Some can be acquired without sexual contact. The most common infections are:

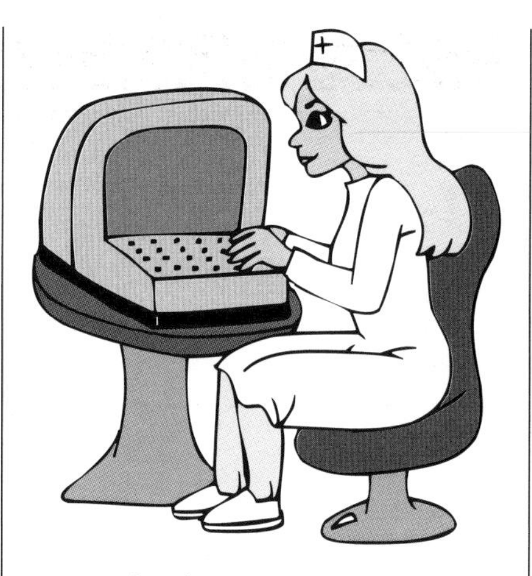

- Chlamydia
- Gonorrhoea
- Genital herpes
- Genital warts
- Non-specific genital infections (NSGIs)
- HIV and AIDS
- Hepatitis B
- Trichomoniasis
- Syphilis

The following are not necessarily transmitted through sexual contact:

- Candidiasis (thrush)
- Pubic lice
- Scabies

■ The above information is from Brook's website: www.brook.org.uk For more contact information, see their details on page 41.

Sexually transmitted diseases in the UK

An overview

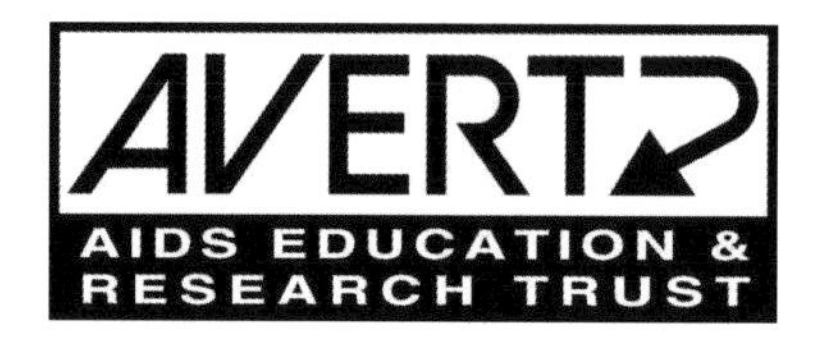

Since 1995, there has been a sustained increase in diagnoses of most STIs (also called STDs) in the UK. Two of the most common STDs have had massive increases. Uncomplicated gonorrhoea increased by 139% between 1995 and 2003. However, between 2002 and 2003 it fell by 3% overall, one of only two STDs to show a reduction in the number of cases.

Cases of genital chlamydia increased by 192% between 1995 and 2003. The increase in the number of chlamydia cases between 2002 and 2003 was 9%, demonstrating that its incidence is continuing to rise, in spite of belated government efforts to fight it. Chlamydia can have serious side-effects, one of which is Pelvic Inflammatory Disease (PID) which can lead to infertility in women. Chlamydia can often be symptomless and therefore people do not come forward to be tested – they may often have no idea that they're infected. In 2003 the government announced a chlamydia screening programme to help diagnose and treat this ever-increasing disease. They recommended that all sexually active women in the UK under the age of 26 should be tested for the infection. This recommendation, however, was not accompanied by any extra funding to allow the testing to take place.

Perhaps that's one reason that since then chlamydia has continued to spread, becoming the most common STD in the UK; the total number of new infections in 2003 was 89,818. It's been the most common STD since 2001, when it overtook genital warts – the first time

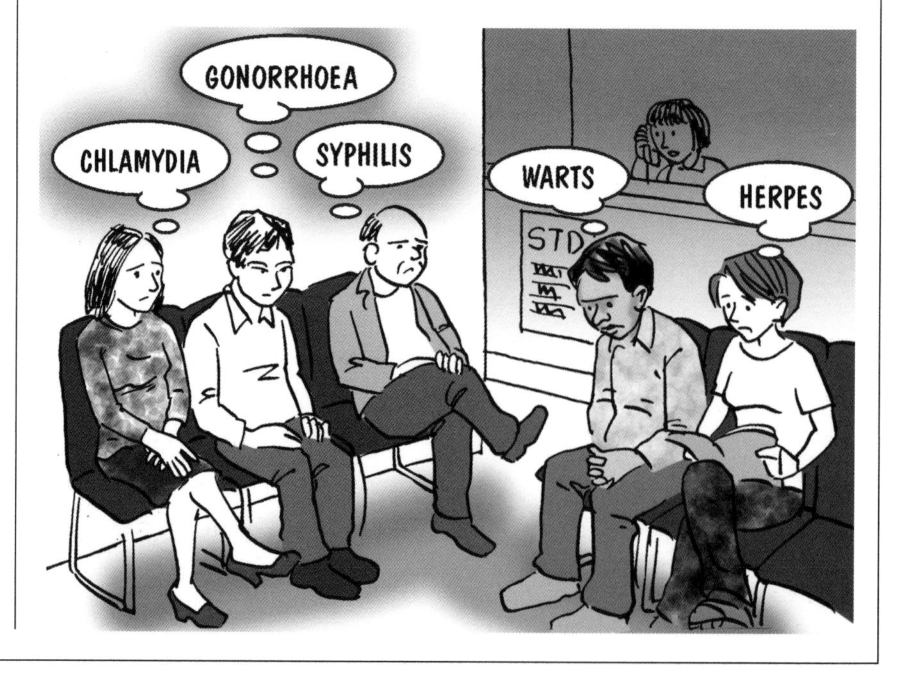

that a bacterial STD had been the most common sexually transmitted infection in the UK.

Syphilis, genital warts and genital herpes

One of the less common STDs in the UK, infectious syphilis, increased by 1058% between 1995 and 2003. This was fuelled by outbreaks between men who have sex with men (MSM) in London, Manchester and Brighton. Though the numbers involved in contracting syphilis are considerably lower than that of chlamydia, it is still a worrying trend, as syphilis can have serious health implications and has been thought for years to be under control in the UK. Cases of genital herpes and genital warts rose by 15% and 27% respectively, between 1995 and 2003.

Who's affected by STDs?

The burden of sexually transmitted infections falls unequally in the population; young heterosexuals, MSM and minority ethnic groups are at increased risk. In 2003, 42% of females with gonorrhoea and 36% of females with genital chlamydial infection were under 20 years of age. 22% of diagnoses of gonorrhoea were in MSM, 53% of which were diagnosed in London. 48% of gonococcal isolates included in the sentinel survey of antibiotic resistant gonorrhoea were seen in women identified as having a black ethnicity.

GUM clinics can't cope

There are 1.5 million attendances at genitourinary medicine clinics in the UK each year, a number which has been growing by at least 15% annually. This increase in people using GUM services has inevitably put pressure on their ability to deal with this number of infections, and has led to delays in waiting times. This pressure on GUM services was highlighted in a House of Commons Health Committee report on sexual health, published in 2003. They said that 'England is currently witnessing a rapid decline in its sexual health . . . sexual health services appear ill-equipped to deal with the crisis that confronts them.' Median waiting times to services are currently around 10-12 days and some services are turning hundreds of people away each week.

United Kingdom STD statistics

Year	Syphilis	Gonorrhoea	Chlamydia	Herpes	Warts
1995	136	10,186	30,794	15,645	55,608
1996	122	12,140	34,136	15,915	59,216
1997	151	12,656	40,583	15,766	63,554
1998	132	12,829	46,155	16,421	64,925
1999	215	15,974	53,783	16,581	66,439
2000	327	21,131	64,800	16,944	66,144
2001	736	22,997	71,967	17,876	68,019
2002	1,232	25,065	82,558	18,432	69,569
2003	1,575	24,039	89,818	17,990	70,883
% change (2002-2003)	28%	-3%	9%	-2%	2%
% change (1995-2003)	1,058%	139%	192%	15%	27%

Source: Avert

Waiting times rise, infections rise

If people are not being treated quickly, this can have inevitable effects on the spread of infection. Factors such as increases in risky sexual behaviour, the greater acceptability of using GUM services and new campaigns to encourage testing have all contributed to the rise seen in new infections of STDs. The rapid increase in bacterial STDs, such as chlamydia, probably reflects a general deterioration in sexual health amongst young people and MSM, although increased testing for genital chlamydia and improved test sensitivity have also contributed.

There are 1.5 million attendances at genitourinary medicine clinics in the UK each year, a number which has been growing by at least 15% annually

STD infection can have grave consequences for an individual's health, and even if it can be successfully treated, is likely to be traumatic. No one wants to be told that they have a serious, often disfiguring sexually transmitted infection, and then be told to come back next week, or the week after. A recent report shows that 28% of all emergency cases were not seen within 48 hours. This is the consequence of the government's advising people to get tested for STDs and then not providing the facilities for them to get help.

The long waiting times for treatment at clinics are increasing the spread of STD epidemics. The worst aspect of the soaring STD levels in this country are that they are entirely preventable, if we had a government that was willing to spend more and to have a frank and open discussion on a subject that it seems still embarrassed to talk about – sexual health.

■ The above information is an extract from AVERT's website which can be found at www.avert.org Alternatively, see page 41 for their address details.

Sex infections rise again

By Debbie Andalo

Sexually transmitted disease in the UK is continuing to increase with a 4% rise in reported cases, according to official figures released 27 July 2004.

The number of new cases of syphilis showed the highest increase between 2002 and 2003 with a rise of 28%, while diagnoses of chlamydia went up by 9% in the same period. There was also a 2% increase in cases of genital warts, the statistics from the Health Protection Agency reveal.

During the same period, however, there was a slight fall of 3% in the number of cases of gonorrhoea, with a 2% drop in the number of new cases of genital herpes.

The chairman of the British Medical Association, James Johnson, condemned the figures. He said: 'Another year, another set of figures and yet more predictions of an impending public health crisis. Well, I've got news for the government, the crisis is here.

'It is a scandal that the service we offer patients today is worse than it was 90 years ago,' he said.

Releasing the figures for England, Wales and Northern Ireland, the HPA chairman, Sir William Stewart, said: 'These are preventable infections and it is a cause of considerable concern that we are still seeing increases in new diagnosis of sexually transmitted infections (STIs) across the UK and unsafe sex is undoubtedly a main contributor to this.'

He accepted that part of the increase reflected more people coming forward for testing because of increased awareness of STIs, but pointed out that gay men and young people generally were most affected.

Dr Angela Robinson, president of the British Association of Sexual Health and HIV, which represents healthcare professionals, said the figures mirrored increased workload at genitourinary medicine (GUM) clinics. She said: 'Prompt access to GUM services for patients is essential if the number of new infections is to be reduced.'

In a statement, the public health minister, Melanie Johnson, said the government had invested £26m in improving access to GUM clinics and developing services. It has also highlighted the risks of STI in its sex lottery campaign which aimed to change sexual behaviour of those most at risk.

The number of new cases of syphilis showed the highest increase between 2002 and 2003 with a rise of 28%, while diagnoses of chlamydia went up by 9% in the same period

Comparison of numbers of new diagnoses between 2002 and 2003 shows:

- Chlamydia increased by 9% (from 82,558 in 2002 to 89,818)
- Syphilis increased by 28% (from 1,232 in 2002 to 1,575)
- Gonorrhoea decreased by 3% (from 25,065 in 2002 to 24,309)
- Genital warts increased by 2% (from 69,569 in 2002 to 70,883)
- Genital herpes decreased by 2% (from 18,432 in 2002 to 17,990)

- Meanwhile the FPA, the charity devoted to sexual health and protecting an individual's reproductive rights, released the results of its own survey which showed that only two new GUM clinics have opened since 2002 and 54% of the existing 256 GUM clinics in the UK were open less than 21 hours a week.

Selected conditions by sex

Summary table of selected conditions and total diagnosis by sex: England, Wales and Northern Ireland,* 1995-2003

Syphilis (Primary & secondary)	1997	1998	1999	2000	2001	2002	2003
Total males	101	88	160	252	633	1,095	1,394
(of which homosexually acquired)	19	23	52	123	362	633	783
Total females	50	44	55	75	103	137	181
Total	**151**	**132**	**215**	**327**	**736**	**1,232**	**1,575**
Gonorrhoea (uncomplicated)	**1997**	**1998**	**1999**	**2000**	**2001**	**2002**	**2003**
Total males	8,602	8,649	10,972	14,725	16,096	17,457	16,841
(of which homosexually acquired)	1,804	1,698	1,842	2,939	3,551	3,376	3,757
Total females	4,054	4,180	5,002	6,406	6,901	7,608	7,468
Total	**12,656**	**12,829**	**15,974**	**21,131**	**22,997**	**25,065**	**24,309**
Chlamydia (uncomplicated)	**1997**	**1998**	**1999**	**2000**	**2001**	**2002**	**2003**
Total males	16,985	19,896	22,962	28,100	31,201	36,234	39,977
(of which homosexually acquired)	357	466	633	990	1,412	1,469	1,793
Total females	23,598	26,259	30,821	36,700	40,766	46,324	49,841
Total	**40,583**	**46,155**	**53,783**	**64,800**	**71,967**	**82,558**	**89,818**
Herpes (first attack)	**1997**	**1998**	**1999**	**2000**	**2001**	**2002**	**2003**
Total males	5,870	6,356	6,302	6,473	6,798	6,841	6,698
(of which homosexually acquired)	337	303	344	400	411	490	474
Total females	9,896	10,065	10,279	10,471	11,078	11,591	11,292
Total	**15,766**	**16,421**	**16,581**	**16,944**	**17,876**	**18,922**	**17,990**
Warts (first attack)	**1997**	**1998**	**1999**	**2000**	**2001**	**2002**	**2003**
Total males	32,679	33,670	34,716	34,847	35,650	36,995	37,458
(of which homosexually acquired)	1,499	1,544	1,608	1,729	1,848	2,056	2,184
Total females	30,875	31,255	31,723	31,297	32,369	32,574	33,425
Total	**63,554**	**64,925**	**66,439**	**66,144**	**68,019**	**69,569**	**70,883**

* UK totals are not presented as 2001 and 2002 data for Scotland are not currently available.

Source: Health Protection Agency, Crown copyright

Sexually transmitted infections

Information from fpa

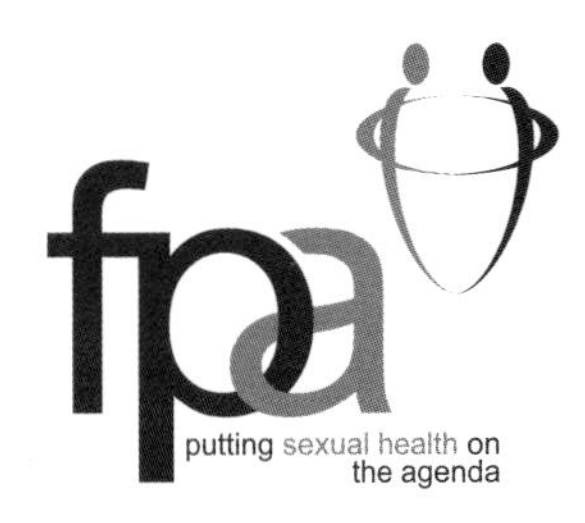

There are at least 25 different sexually transmitted infections. Below is some information about eight of the most common STIs:

Chlamydia

What is chlamydia?
Chlamydia is a bacteria that can infect the genitals, urethra and rectum of men and women, but may also affect the throat and eyes.

How is it passed on?
It is passed on by unprotected vaginal, oral or anal sex, when sharing sex toys, or by a mother to her baby at birth.

Signs and symptoms
About 50% of men and 70% of women with chlamydia show no symptoms at all. Often symptoms are very mild and go unnoticed, but typical signs of infection with chlamydia experienced by men or women include:

- Unusual discharge from the penis or vagina.
- Pain when passing urine.
- Bleeding between periods.
- Testicular pain or swelling.
- Pain during sex.
- Low abdominal pain.

Tests and treatment

- Usually a swab is taken from the vagina or tip of the penis and a sample of urine is taken. The swab might feel a bit uncomfortable but is quick and should not be painful.
- Chlamydia is easily treated with antibiotics. To avoid re-infection, sexual partners should also be treated.
- If untreated, chlamydia can spread to other reproductive organs causing serious health problems such as pelvic inflammatory disease, ectopic pregnancy and infertility.

Gonorrhoea

What is gonorrhoea?
Gonorrhoea is a bacteria that mainly infects the genitals, urethra, rectum and throat of men and women.

How is it passed on?
It is passed on by unprotected vaginal, oral or anal sex, sharing sex toys, or by a mother to her baby at birth.

Signs and symptoms
About 10% of men and 50% of women with gonorrhoea show no symptoms. Symptoms can be mild and go unnoticed, but typical signs of infection include:

- Unusual discharge from the penis or vagina that can be thin or watery, or yellow or green.
- Pain when passing urine.
- Possible irritation or discharge from the anus.
- Lower abdominal pain.
- Pain or tenderness in the testicles.

Tests and treatment

- Usually a swab is taken from the vagina or tip of the penis and a sample of urine may be taken.

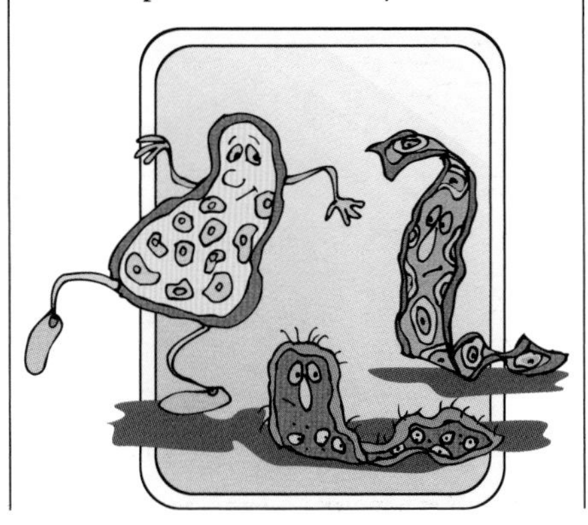

The swab may feel a bit uncomfortable but should not be painful.
- Gonorrhoea is easily treated with antibiotics. To avoid re-infection, sexual partners should also be treated.
- If untreated, gonorrhoea can infect other reproductive organs in men and women and lead to serious health problems such as pelvic inflammatory disease or ectopic pregnancy, which can affect fertility.

Genital warts

What are genital warts?
Genital warts are caused by the human papilloma virus (HPV). This virus can affect the hands, feet and genital area. This information is about genital warts.

How are they passed on?
Genital warts are passed on through unprotected vaginal or anal sex, by sharing sex toys or direct skin-to-skin genital contact.

Signs and symptoms
Not everyone with the virus will develop visible warts. When warts are present they are usually painless but may cause some inflammation.

- Warts can be flat, smooth, small bumps or larger cauliflower-like lumps that occur on their own or in groups.
- In men, they can appear anywhere around the urethra, penis, scrotum or anus. They can also appear inside the anus.
- In women, they can appear anywhere around the vulva and anus, and also inside the vagina or anus, or on the cervix.

Tests and treatment

- Usually warts can be seen with the naked eye. If they are suspected, but not obvious, the

area is painted with a special solution to make them more visible.
- Warts are easy to treat, but more than one treatment may be needed.
- Treatment can include covering the warts with a chemical lotion or cream, freezing them off or removing them by laser treatment or surgery.
- Genital warts do not cause any serious health problems but the virus always remains in the body. No treatment can remove the virus completely.
- Some types of the wart virus are linked to changes in cervical cells which could lead to cervical cancer. These changes can take many years, so it is important women have regular cervical smears, whether or not they have had genital warts.
- IMPORTANT: never self-treat genital warts with over-the-counter remedies

Genital Herpes

What is genital herpes?

Genital herpes is caused by the herpes simplex virus. There are two types of the virus, which can affect the mouth and nose (known as cold sores) or the genital and anal area, fingers or hands. This information is about genital herpes.

How is it passed on?

It is passed on by unprotected vaginal, oral or anal sex, through sharing sex toys or through direct skin-to-skin genital contact.

Signs and symptoms

Often symptoms don't show or are very mild and go unnoticed, but typical signs of infection with the virus include:
- Blisters on or in the vagina, cervix, urethra, rectum, anus or penis that leave painful sores when they burst.
- Tingling or itching feeling in the affected area.
- Flu-like symptoms such as swollen glands, backache and headache.

Tests and treatment
- A swab is taken from one of the sores and a sample of urine may be taken. The swab may feel uncomfortable but should not be painful.
- Left untreated, the symptoms may last about 2-3 weeks. Genital herpes does not cause serious health problems and it doesn't affect fertility.
- If the infection reoccurs, symptoms are usually milder. The virus always remains in the body and no treatment can remove it completely.
- Some people find that different things can trigger an attack. These include stress, tiredness, illness, alcohol and smoking. Avoiding these helps reduce the number of attacks.

More information about herpes can be obtained from the Herpes Viruses Association on 020 7609 9061, website www.herpes.org.uk

> ***There are at least 25 different sexually transmitted infections***

Syphilis

What is syphilis?

Syphilis is a bacteria that infects the vulva, urethra, or cervix in women and the penis or foreskin in men.

How is it passed on?

It is passed on through unprotected vaginal, oral or anal sex, by sharing sex toys, direct skin-to-skin contact with someone who has syphilis sores

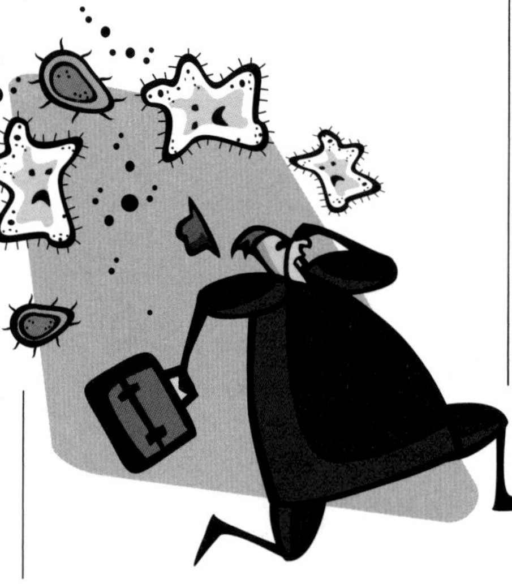

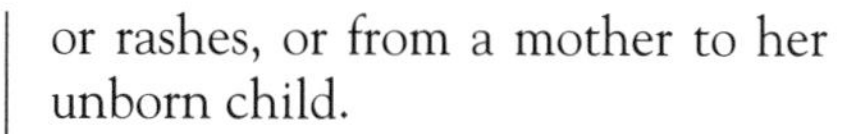

or rashes, or from a mother to her unborn child.

Signs and symptoms

Sometimes symptoms go unnoticed, but typical signs of first-stage syphilis infection include:
- One or more painless sores on or in the genital area of men and women which can last around 3-4 weeks.

If the infection is not treated, second-stage syphilis can occur and typical symptoms include:
- A rash over the whole body or in patches.
- Flu-like symptoms such as swollen glands, tiredness, headache and sore throat.
- Flat, wart-like growths on the genitals.

Tests and treatments
- A swab is taken from one of the sores and blood and urine samples will be taken. The swab might be a bit uncomfortable but should not be painful.
- Syphilis is easily treated with antibiotics. To avoid re-infection, sexual partners should also be treated.
- Pregnant women can be treated safely with no risk to the unborn baby.
- Left untreated, syphilis can have very serious consequences over time to all the major organs in the body and this damage can be fatal.

Trichomonas vaginalis

What is Trichomonas vaginalis?

Trichomonas vaginalis is an infection caused by a microscopic parasite found in the vagina and urethra in both women and men.

How is it passed on?

It is passed on through unprotected vaginal, oral or anal sex, possibly by sharing sex toys, or from a mother to her baby at birth.

Signs and symptoms

Sometimes there are no symptoms, or they are so mild they go unnoticed.

Typical signs of infection include:
- A change in vaginal discharge: this may increase,

become thinner, frothy or change in smell.
- A discharge from the penis.
- Inflammation, soreness or itching in and around the vagina.
- Pain on passing urine in both men and women.
- Pain on having sex.

Tests and treatment
- Usually a swab is taken from the urethra, vagina or tip of the penis. This might feel a bit uncomfortable but is quick and should not be painful.
- A sample of urine may be taken.
- Trichomonas vaginalis is easily treated with antibiotics. To avoid re-infection, sexual partners should also be treated.
- If left untreated it doesn't cause any serious health problems.

Scabies and pubic lice

What are scabies and pubic lice?
Scabies and pubic lice are caused by tiny mites or lice. In scabies the mites can occur in any part of the body, but are often seen under the skin in creases such as under the arms, underneath the buttocks, on the hands and wrists, or on the genitals.

Pubic lice live in coarse body hair such as pubic hair, chest and underarm hair. They sometimes live in eyebrows or eyelashes but not on head hair.

How are they passed on?
Scabies is passed on through close physical skin contact. It can also be sexually transmitted, but this is less common.

Pubic lice are usually passed on through sexual contact. They can also be passed on through close physical contact.

Signs and symptoms
- Scabies causes an itchy rash in the body's skin creases, which may also be accompanied by tiny spots.
- Pubic lice causes itchy skin and black powder appears in the underwear caused by mite droppings. White eggs can be found on affected hair.

Tests and treatment
- For both scabies and pubic lice, the skin will be examined and a skin flake may be taken to test for mites or lice.
- Scabies and pubic lice are easily treated with a special lotion or shampoo. These kill the mites or lice and their eggs. To avoid re-infection, close contacts or sexual partners should also be treated.
- Neither scabies or pubic lice cause any long-term health problems.

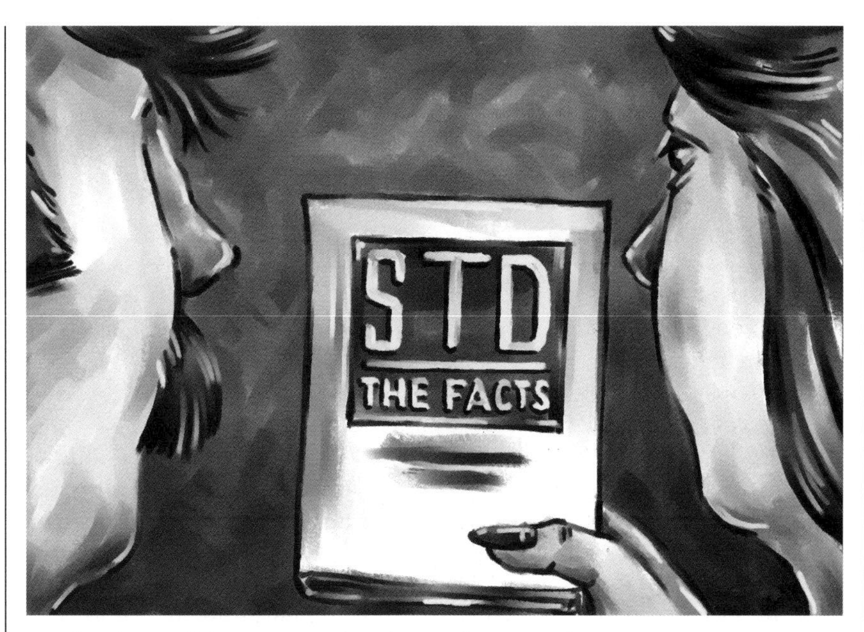

HIV and AIDS

What is HIV?
HIV stands for the Human Immunodeficiency Virus and affects men and women. The virus damages the body's immune system so that over time it becomes vulnerable to illness and infections.

What is AIDS?
AIDS is caused by HIV. When a person has AIDS it means their immune system is very weak and they have developed certain infections or cancers. These can be fatal.

How is it passed on?
HIV is mainly passed on in the following ways:
- By unprotected vaginal or anal sex.
- By sharing needles or syringes when injecting drugs.
- A pregnant woman with HIV can pass it on to her baby during birth, although there is now a very effective treatment to help prevent this. HIV can also be passed on through breastfeeding.

Signs and symptoms
- A flu-like illness may occur shortly after getting infected with HIV, but most people don't notice they have become infected.
- Symptoms vary from person to person and occur when the immune system is so damaged that other infections begin to cause health problems.

Tests and treatment
- The only way to establish if a person has the virus is for them to have an HIV test.
- After a discussion about the test and the consequences of the result, a sample of blood will be taken and tested. It is necessary to wait three months after infection might have occurred before doing the HIV test.
- There is no cure for HIV. However, drugs are available to slow down the damage that HIV does to the immune system. People who are HIV positive can now stay healthy for many years with anti-HIV drugs.

If you would like information about other sexually transmitted infections you can telephone the fpa helpline on 0845 310 1334 or visit www.ssha.info

■ The above information was based on evidence and medical opinion available at the time of printing and is from fpa's website: www.fpa.org.uk

Young, free and infectious

Rates of sexually transmitted diseases are rising alarmingly; overworked clinics are turning patients away; and still young people aren't getting the message about unprotected sex. Julie Wheelwright on Britain's teenage sexual health crisis

In her navy blue track suit, Jasmine crosses her legs and shifts her gym bag more comfortably on to her lap. She sits opposite Dr Emma Fox, the consultant who runs Bridge, a pioneering sexual health clinic for under-20s at Guy's Hospital in south London. Jasmine explains tentatively that her contraceptive pill has been causing irregular bleeding and she doesn't know why. Fox notes her symptoms and runs through a list of questions. 'Is this a regular sexual partner?'; 'Is he from another country?'; 'Do you use condoms?'; 'Have you had any other sexual partners?'

At the last question, Jasmine gives a wobbly smile. This is her first boyfriend and she was sexually inexperienced before they got together. Fox assesses that her patient is low-risk for HIV but suggests running a screen for syphilis and gonorrhea because either of these infections could explain the bleeding. Her next patient, another young woman, had unprotected sex with a stranger in March and is concerned that she might have put herself at risk of HIV or chlamydia. She just wants to be 'totally safe', and Fox refers her for testing in another room.

The need for a clinic aimed at young people could not be more stark. Britain has the worst sexual health in Europe and the boroughs of Lambeth, Southwark and Lewisham, in south London, have the highest rates of sexually transmitted infections (STIs) in the country. The incidence of chlamydia has risen by 50% in teenagers in the past three years alone. Fox, who has headed Bridge since its opening in February this year, says an estimated 15% of her patients have this infection, which can be asymptomatic and lead to infertility in women if untreated. These south London boroughs also have a quarter of all UK cases of gonorrhea.

By Julie Wheelwright

'Having more services isn't the answer to improving teenage sexual health,' says Fox. 'The government has got the right idea with strategies that recognise the link between poverty, social exclusion and poor sexual health, but changing things is actually quite difficult.' The young people who attend Bridge, however, are fortunate because they can avoid the queues and waiting lists that affect genito-urinary medicine clinics throughout the country. As STI rates soar, with cases of chlamydia having increased by 140% between 1996 and 2002, and HIV diagnoses by 200%, clinics are burdened with huge increases in their caseloads.

As patients are turned away from overcrowded clinics before they can be diagnosed or treated, they run the risk of infecting others

Even worse, as patients are turned away from overcrowded clinics before they can be diagnosed or treated, they run the risk of infecting others; studies suggest that approximately a third of patients with symptomatic STIs continue to have sexual intercourse. The consequences can be devastating. Rebecca, 23, slept with a former boyfriend who claimed he hadn't been with anyone else since their split. 'He wanted to break it off so he could have told me anything and I would have had him back,' she says. 'We slept together and then I started having really painful cramping, even when it wasn't my period.' Rebecca's test proved positive for chlamydia and after a course of antibiotics, she got the all-clear.

Rebecca regards herself as fortunate because an untreated STI can lead to chronic illness or permanent damage. 'It can take a lot of courage to turn up to one of these places and if you're told to come back in six weeks, that person might not come back,' says Jan Barlow, chief executive of the Brook advisory service. 'We certainly hear cases of people being turned away at GUM clinics.' Although the problem is

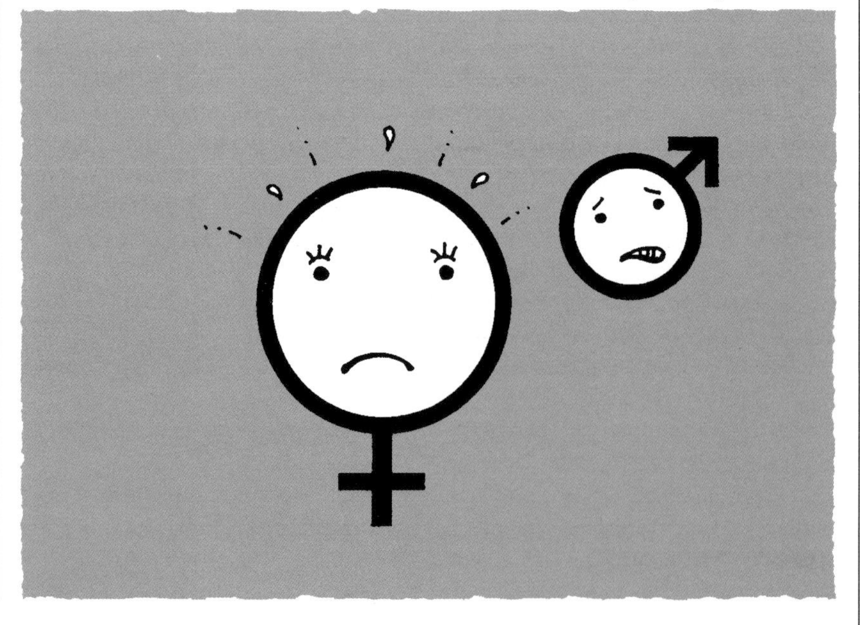

more acute for young people, with women under 20 having the highest rates of gonorrhea and chlamydia, all sexual health services are currently under pressure.

Bill, 37, describes his experience of visiting a walk-in clinic in east London that was so crowded, people were sitting on the floors and in the corridors. A year ago, Bill, suspecting the symptoms of an infection, headed to a clinic near work for treatment and found the door locked. 'I got there in good time but found a sign saying, "Due to too many patients, we have closed the clinic early,"' he says. 'The trouble was that I was going to eastern Europe for a 10-day holiday so I couldn't just come back the next day.' A few days into his trip, Bill developed a raging sore throat and took an antibiotic to clear up the symptoms. 'I knew I was in deep shit,' he says. 'But what do you do? I was moving around and wasn't in one place so I foolishly decided to treat myself.'

The symptoms cleared up. But a few weeks later, Bill began to have painful swelling in his tendons, chest pains and was becoming breathless. 'The doctors kept telling me they didn't think anything was wrong with me and wanted to prescribe anti-depressants.' A few months later, he developed stiff joints but was told he was too young to have arthritis and it was nearly a year before he was finally diagnosed with Reiter's syndrome, a condition caused by untreated gonorrhea.

Bill admits that he had unprotected sex while he was on holiday, a mistake that Ann, aged 29, also made. 'Earlier this year I split up with my husband and went on holiday to Spain. It was the usual thing of meeting a guy, having had too much to drink and I didn't think anything of it until I got home and talked to a girlfriend.' Although Ann had no symptoms of an infection, her friend suggested she get tested. So, one lunchtime, she went to a walk-in clinic. She was shocked to discover that she had tested positive for chlamydia. 'I would never make the same mistake again,' she says. 'Some people think it only affects stupid 16-year-olds but it affects everyone.'

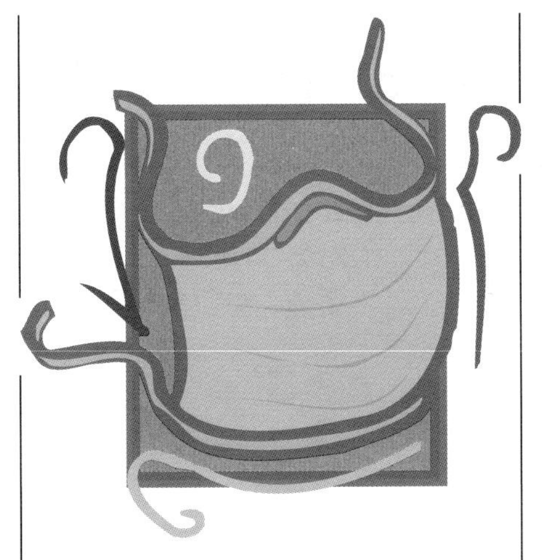

In fact, the risk of contracting an STI has increased as people have more partners and engage in riskier sexual behaviour. 'Condom use has increased but it hasn't kept pace with the unsafe sex that people are having,' says Dr Patrick French, who runs the Mortimer Market Centre clinic at University College, London. 'People are having sex at a younger age and there are more overlapping relationships and partners. Young people are crying out for more support about the message out there that starting sex early is what's expected.'

Sexual health professionals all seem to agree that destigmatising sexual health and starting sex education at an early age are vitally important to curbing the dramatic rise in infections. With the government's planning and priority framework for health expected soon, the Terrence Higgins Trust is lobbying to make sexual health a priority while the Independent Advisory Group on Sexual Health and HIV is pushing for work on prevention.

There are cutting-edge projects already operating in Lambeth. Dr Claire Gerada, a local GP in south London, has been visiting primary schools in the borough for the past five years, teaching children how to negotiate relationships with their peers, how to resist peer pressure and what changes their bodies go through during puberty. Gerada says she often visits schools where the detailed questions the children ask suggest they are already sexually active.

In a year-six class on a Monday morning, a mixed class of girls and boys sit quietly, their hands folded, their desks neat. Gerada is asking the children what they know about puberty. They eagerly raise their hands, desperate to give answers. 'Boys get sperm', 'Sometimes your voice breaks', 'Girls' hips widen'. One girl asks how far a penis can travel up a vagina and another asks if you can get pregnant before you've started your periods. When Gerada asks why condoms are important, a girl in plaits says calmly, 'Because it stops spreading diseases.'

Afterwards the children tell me confidently that they think these lessons, which they started in reception, will affect the choices they make once they leave primary school. 'I really do think it will change the way I think about sex and relationships in high school,' says Emma, 11. 'I won't just jump straight into things.' Her classmate Lawrence agrees. 'These lessons are preparing us for secondary school because if we talk about sexual relationships now, we have an idea of what's going to happen there. It's a good start for us.'

French, who may have these children walking through his clinic doors in a few years, agrees that the key to combating STIs lies in early education. 'In countries where children get sexual and relationship education from age seven, they start having sex later, they're much more grown up and responsible,' he says. 'Now we're at a time when people are more open, we need to keep pushing on that open door.'

■ Some of the names in this article have been changed.

■ The following correction was printed in the *Guardian*'s Corrections and clarifications column, Saturday 10 July 2004.

We say below that Reiter's syndrome, also known as reactive arthritis, is 'a condition caused by untreated gonorrhea'. That is not its only cause. According to the Arthritis Foundation, the exact cause is unknown, but about 75% of the those with the tendency to develop it have a special gene marker. Reiter's can develop following an infection in the intestines or genital or urinary tract. See www.arthritis.org for more details.

Sexual health check-ups

Information from www.aidsmap.com

for hiv information

nam

Why check-ups are important

In recent years there has been a substantial increase in the number of sexually transmitted infections in the UK, most notably the bacterial infections syphilis, gonorrhoea and chlamydia. Many of the people diagnosed with syphilis have been HIV-positive gay men.

Why check-ups are important

If you are sexually active there's a chance that you can pick up a sexually transmitted infection.

Some of these infections can mean that you have an increased risk of passing HIV onto somebody else during unprotected anal, oral or vaginal sex.

Sexually transmitted infections don't always cause symptoms, so a check-up and tests are often needed to tell if you have an infection.

Sexual health check-ups provide an opportunity to test you for, and vaccinate you against, the liver viruses hepatitis A and B. Hepatitis C seems to be more readily passed on sexually to and by people with HIV, and you can also be tested to see if you have been infected with this virus.

Condoms and lubricants are available free of charge from sexual health clinics.

Where to go

Most HIV clinics have a sexual health clinic attached. What's more an increasing number of the large HIV clinics are starting to offer sexual health screens to their patients as part of their routine HIV care.

What to expect

All tests and treatment offered by NHS sexual health clinics are free of charge. You can choose which sexual health clinic you go to – you do not have to go to the one in your local area or the one associated with your HIV clinic.

Some sexual health clinics operate on a walk-in basis. If you go to a walk-in clinic be prepared for a long wait. If your chosen clinic operates an appointment system, then you may have to wait days or even weeks for the next available appointment. If you have symptoms make sure that you say so when making your appointment, as there may well be a number of emergency appointments available allowing you to be seen more promptly.

Sexually transmitted infections don't always cause symptoms, so a check-up and tests are often needed to tell if you have an infection

When you go to the clinic, you will be asked to register. Your details will remain confidential.

First of all you will be seen by a doctor, who will ask you about the kind of sex you have been having, ask you if you have any symptoms and examine you. Try to answer the doctor's questions as fully and truthfully as possible – this will ensure that you have the most appropriate tests. Also make sure to tell the doctor if you are taking any medication, including anti-HIV drugs, or are allergic to any medicines.

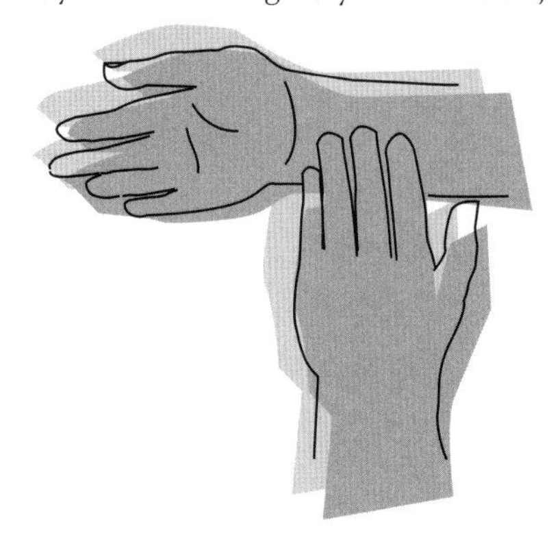

You will then be seen by a nurse for the tests the doctor thinks you need to have. Men can expect to have at least one swab taken from the tip of the penis, and women at least one swab from the vagina. It's important not to pass urine for at least two hours before you go to the clinic. If you do, your swabs might not show if you have an infection. If you have had anal and/or oral sex, swabs will be taken from the anus and/or throat. It's likely that blood samples will be taken to check for syphilis and, if you are a gay man or injecting drug user, for hepatitis A, B, and C.

If you have sores on your genitals these may also be swabbed to check to see if you have herpes.

You will be asked to provide a urine sample.

Some of the test results will be available immediately, but you will be asked to call back a week or so later to get some other results.

If you do have an infection, you will be given treatment. You will be asked to return after you have finished taking your treatment to make sure that it has worked.

If you have an infection you will be given an opportunity to see a Health Adviser, who can give you information about safer sex and how to protect your own and other people's sexual health. They will also ask you to help them, where possible or practicable, to contact your sexual partners so they can be tested and treated too. Where appropriate, Health Advisers can provide referrals to other services.

If you have genital warts you will be asked to come in regularly for treatment which will be provided by a nurse without an appointment.

■ The above information is from Aid map's website which can be found at www.aidsmap.com

Patients wait six weeks to visit sex disease clinics

By James Meikle, Health Correspondent

People with sexually transmitted infections are having to wait up to six weeks for an appointment at specialist clinics – a key factor in the rise of the diseases, health campaigners said 27 July 2004.

They accused ministers of failing to make the crisis a priority as the government's Health Protection Agency revealed that new diagnoses in England, Wales and Northern Ireland rose by 4% last year to more than 708,000.

Ministers tried to claim credit for a slowing in the rate of increase compared with most of the past decade.

There has been a 57% rise since the mid-1990s, but there were still some huge annual increases in particular infections.

Syphilis cases, still comparatively rare, rose by 28% in a year and by 1058% since 1995, and there was a 9% annual rise in chlamydia, up 192% since the mid-1990s.

Increasingly risky sexual behaviour and delays in treatments have prompted demands for improved access to clinics, substantial extra funding and better sex education, especially for young people and gay men.

The Family Planning Association's chief executive, Anne Weymann, said: 'Treating sexually transmitted infections and their consequences costs the NHS an estimated £1bn a year.

'Fast access to treatment is essential to prevent the spread of infection and makes economic sense, yet waiting times are as long as six weeks.'

Surveys showed that more than half of those questioned did not know they could go to clinics without consulting their GPs, and more than 80% did not know NHS prescriptions linked to treatments were free.

A survey of clinics found that 54% of the 256 across Britain advertised opening times of less than 21 hours a week. While one in five had added sessions, one in six had cut them.

Just two new clinics had opened in the last two years.

Ms Weymann said: 'The secrecy and the stigma that surround STIs is a threat to the nation's health.'

'Fast access to treatment is essential to prevent the spread of infection and makes economic sense, yet waiting times are as long as six weeks'

Angela Robinson, the president of the British Association of Sexual Health and HIV, said a third of patients were waiting more than two weeks, when there should be a 48-hour target for access to clinics.

Nick Partridge, the chief executive of the Terrence Higgins Trust, said the figures were an indictment of NHS inaction in making sexual health a priority.

The figures, revealed by the government's Health Protection Agency, did not detail HIV infection or clinic waiting times, issues expected to be addressed by the chief medical officer, Sir Liam Donaldson, 28 July 2004.

Kevin Fenton, the head of the agency's HIV and STI department, said: 'The longer you are waiting with an STI, there is a good evidence to suggest that people don't usually stop having sex.'

Some infection rates, for instance for gonorrhoea, fell last year and results vary from region to region, with most infections in London and the north-west of England.

Melanie Johnson, the public health minister, said the government was increasing capacity in sexual health services and had already invested £28m to reduce waiting times and improve access.

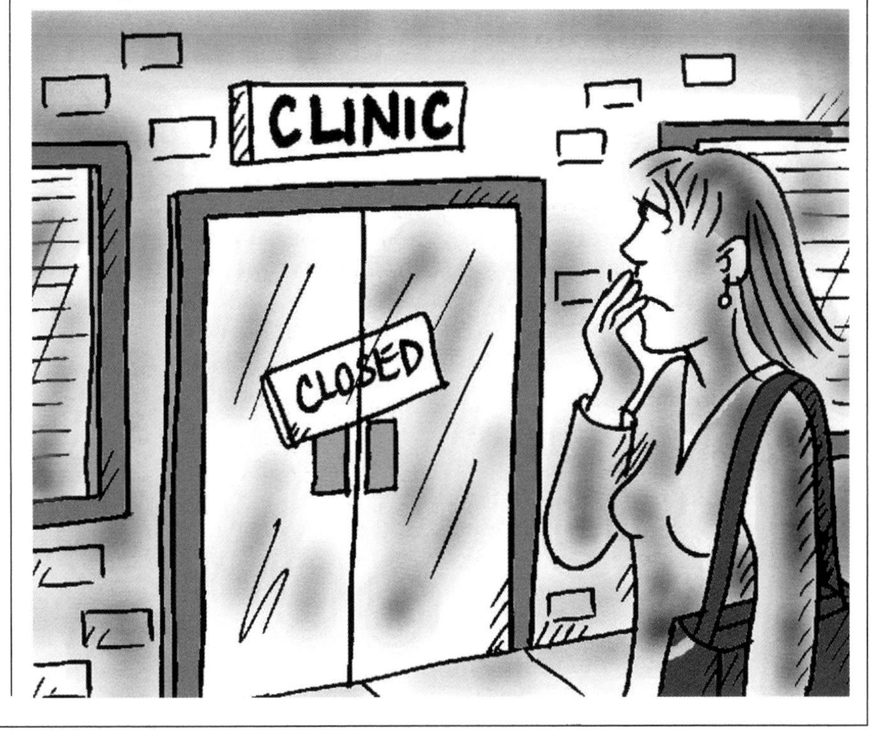

Unprotected sex

Information from www.aidsmap.com

Unprotected sex is any form of anal, oral or vaginal sexual contact which does not involve the use of a male or female condom or similar barrier. Many sexually transmitted infections (STIs) can be passed on via unprotected sex. Unprotected penetrative (the insertion of the penis into the body of another person) anal and vaginal sex carries the greatest risk of STIs, however, infections can also be transmitted through oral sex (mouth to genitals), and oral-anal sex (mouth to anus), also called 'rimming'. For oral sex, some people choose flavoured condoms. For anal sex, it is very important that condoms are used with plenty of water-based lubricant, you should never use oil-based lubricants as these weaken the rubber in condoms. Spermicides with nonoxynol-9 should be avoided as these cause irritation making it more likely that HIV or an STI can be passed on.

Unprotected sex with HIV-negative and untested people

If you are HIV-positive, using condoms during sex with people who know that they are HIV-negative or are unsure of their HIV status will protect them against HIV and protect both of you from STIs. Even if you are taking anti-HIV drugs and have an undetectable viral load in your blood, you may still have enough virus in your semen or vaginal fluids to pass on HIV. You should also be aware that in some countries including certain states of the USA you are legally required to disclose your HIV status to sexual partners. In the UK people have recently been sent to prison after infecting their sexual partners with HIV.

Sex with other HIV-positive people

If you are HIV-positive and having sex with another person who is also HIV-positive, many health promotion experts and HIV and sexual health doctors will recommend that you still continue to use condoms because:

- There is a risk of pregnancy as a consequence of unprotected vaginal sex between men and women. There is a risk of transmission to the baby, when an HIV-positive man has unprotected sex with an HIV-negative woman who is pregnant or breastfeeding. See the fact sheets 31, *Mother to Baby Transmission*, and 54, *Pregnancy and Contraception*, for more information.
- There is growing evidence that it is possible to be super-infected with a new strain or strains of HIV, which may either be more aggressive than or resistant to anti-HIV drugs. This could lead to the failure of treatments that might otherwise have been effective. This applies to both men and women.
- Unprotected sex puts you at risk of other sexually transmitted infections. This applies to both men and women.

Bacterial STIs, such as gonorrhoea and chlamydia, can be treated just as easily and successfully in most people with HIV as in people who are HIV-negative, provided that they are diagnosed and treated. Failure to get prompt treatment can lead to infertility and in some cases damage to the internal organs. Syphilis, particularly in people with severely damaged immune systems, can be harder to diagnose and cure and can be more aggressive when the immune system is damaged. There have been syphilis outbreaks, particularly amongst gay men, across western Europe and north America in the past few years and gay men with HIV have been disproportionately affected. In eastern Europe, and much of the rest of the world, syphilis predominately affects heterosexuals and is also linked to increased risk of HIV infection, along with other treatable ulcerating diseases such as chancroid and donovanosis.

There are also viral STIs. Genital herpes and genital warts are not curable, even in people who are HIV-negative. Although both these infections will respond to treatment, they can reoccur and can be harder to control if you have a severely damaged immune system. Genital herpes is linked to an increased risk of HIV transmission, especially when

Exposure category of HIV infection

Exposure category of HIV infections diagnosed in the United Kingdom, 1998-2002

Year of	Homo/ bisexual men	Heterosexual men and women	Injecting drug users	Mother to infant	Blood/blood products	Other/ undetermined[1]	Total (100%)
1998	1355	1160	130	94	10	65	2814
1999	1347	1427	112	82	21	78	3067
2000	1498	1981	109	102	23	107	3820
2001[2]	1714	2829	128	82	25	196	4974
2002[2]	1617	3152	98	99	25	551	5542
Total	7531	10549	577	459	104	997	20217

1 The proportion with route of infection undetermined is always higher for the most recent year because of the time needed to complete follow-up.
2 Numbers will rise for recent years, as further reports are received.

Source: HIV/AIDS Reports. Reports received by the end of June 2003. 'Renewing the focus', Health Protection Agency, November 2003. Crown copyright.

ulcers are present. Some strains of the virus which cause genital warts have been linked with the development of genital cervical and anal cancers.

The liver viruses hepatitis A and B and (less easily) C can also be passed on sexually and can be more complicated in people with HIV. Hepatitis can cause liver damage which can limit HIV treatment options and make you very unwell in its own right. There are vaccines for hepatitis A and B (but not C), which should be available at your HIV treatment centre. Gay men in particular are advised to be vaccinated against hepatitis A and B. After you have been vaccinated it is important to have your immunity to hepatitis A and B checked regularly, as the vaccines do not offer permanent protection.

Some of the opportunistic infections which affect people with HIV can be passed on through sex. Karposi's sarcoma is thought to be passed on sexually through a form of herpes virus. Both HIV-positive and negative people can be affected by gut infections such as Giardia, amoebas (small parasites which live in the gut and cause diarrhoea), cryptosporidium and microsporidium which can be passed on through oral-anal contact or any sexual activity which leads to contaminated faeces getting into the mouth. These infections can cause very severe diarrhoea which is particularly serious in people with badly damaged immune systems.

Having an active, untreated STI increases the amount of HIV in the genital fluids, making HIV easier to pass on if you have unprotected sex. It is recommended that all sexually active people have regular sexual health check-ups. Many HIV treatment centres have sexual health clinics attached, which in the UK offer free and confidential testing and treatment.

■ The above information is from Aid map's website which can be found at www.aidsmap.com

Men and sexual health

More men see sexual health as an issue for them too

A growing number of men regard sexual health as something that concerns them too, Jan Barlow, Chief Executive of Brook, said 29 September 2004, commenting on new figures on the use of NHS Contraceptive Services in England, published by the Department of Health.

Welcoming the figures, which show an overall increase of 14% in the number of men attending clinics, Jan Barlow said:

'It used to be the case that sexual health wasn't even on most men's radar screens, but now the message that this isn't just a women's issue is clearly beginning to get through.

'In recent years more information has been made available on how to prevent sexually transmitted infections as well as unplanned pregnancy. It's encouraging that as a result more men of all ages are beginning to seek information and advice on a range of sexual health issues.

'The even sharper increase in the number of men under the age of 25 who contacted Brook in the same period suggests that young men are particularly aware of the risk of sexually transmitted infections.

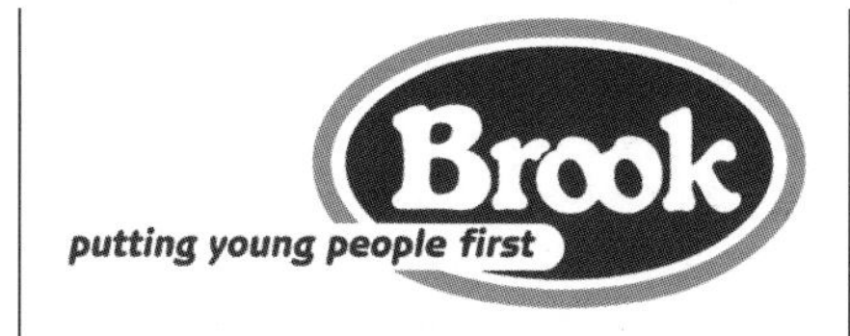

Brook's continuing work to tailor services to the needs of young men is having a real impact.'

The number of male clients under the age of 25 who contacted Brook Centres went up by 30% in 2003-2004, and there was an even more marked increase in the younger age groups, with under 16s increasing by 41% and under 18s increasing by 37%.

Figures show an overall increase of 14% in the number of men attending clinics

Jan also welcomed the increase in the number of NHS family planning clinics for young people, which has tripled since 1994-1995, according the report published 29 September 2004. She added:

'We know from the young people contacting us through our helpline, online and text services that there is a very real need for free and confidential information and advice about sexual health. It is absolutely essential that there is continued investment in clinics set up to meet the needs of young people if we are to see a drop in rates of sexually transmitted infections and unplanned teenage pregnancies.'

■ Brook is the country's leading provider of free, confidential sexual health advice and contraception to young people under 25. The charity has 40 years' experience of providing impartial and confidential sexual health advice and services to young people through a national network of 17 centres across the UK. Each year Brook provides more than 100,000 young people with professional advice from specially trained doctors, nurses, counsellors and outreach and information workers.

Young people can call Brook free and in confidence on 0800 0185 023 or by online enquiry via Ask Brook at www.brook.org.uk

HIV facts

Information from the Terrence Higgins Trust

What is HIV?

HIV is short for Human Immunodeficiency Virus. HIV attacks the body's immune system, making it hard to fight off infections. HIV particularly attacks the white blood cells called CD4 cells, which set the immune system in motion when infections enter the body. HIV infects CD4 cells and uses them to make new copies of HIV which go on to infect more cells. The lower a person's CD4 count, the weaker their immune system will be.

What is AIDS?

AIDS stands for Acquired Immune Deficiency Syndrome. When a person's immune system has been damaged he or she is open to other illnesses, especially infections (e.g. tuberculosis and pneumonia) and cancers, many of which would not normally be a threat. Before effective treatments, if someone with HIV got one of these illnesses the person was said to have AIDS. However, it is no longer a widely-used term. Doctors may instead call this 'late stage' or 'advanced HIV infection'.

How is HIV passed on?

For someone to become infected, a sufficient amount of HIV must get into their blood. The body fluids which contain enough HIV to infect someone are blood, semen, vaginal fluids including menstrual blood, and breast milk.

Saliva, sweat and urine do not contain enough virus to infect someone. HIV cannot pass through intact external skin, or through the air like a cold or flu virus.

The main routes of transmission in the UK are:

- Through sex without a condom – HIV can pass from one person to another through unprotected anal or vaginal sex.

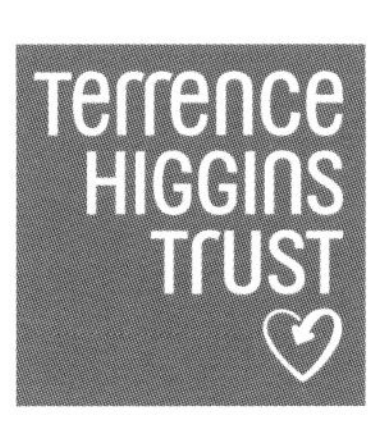

There is only a small risk of transmission through oral sex.

- Through injecting drug use – HIV can be passed on by using needles or syringes that someone with HIV has already used.
- From mother to baby – a pregnant woman may transmit the virus to her baby before or during birth, or HIV can be passed on during breastfeeding.
- Through organ transplant, blood transfusion or blood products – before it was known that donated blood might contain HIV, many people with haemophilia became infected through receiving contaminated blood products. However since 1985, all blood and tissue donations in the UK have been screened for HIV and all blood products are now treated to destroy any HIV which may be present.

How does the HIV test work?

The most commonly used test is an HIV antibody test. Antibodies are produced by the body in response to the presence of HIV, and this test looks for those antibodies.

What is the window period?

When someone becomes infected with HIV, it can take up to three months for their immune system to produce enough antibodies to show up on an HIV test (although in a few cases it can take up to six months) – this gap is known as the window period or seroconversion. Because the HIV test looks for antibodies, taking an HIV test less than three months after possibly getting infected might not give an accurate result. However, throughout the window period, the infected person has enough virus in the blood, breast milk or sexual fluids to infect another person even though it won't show on a test.

Can you treat HIV?

There is no vaccine or cure for HIV. However, anti-HIV drugs are available, and taking a combination

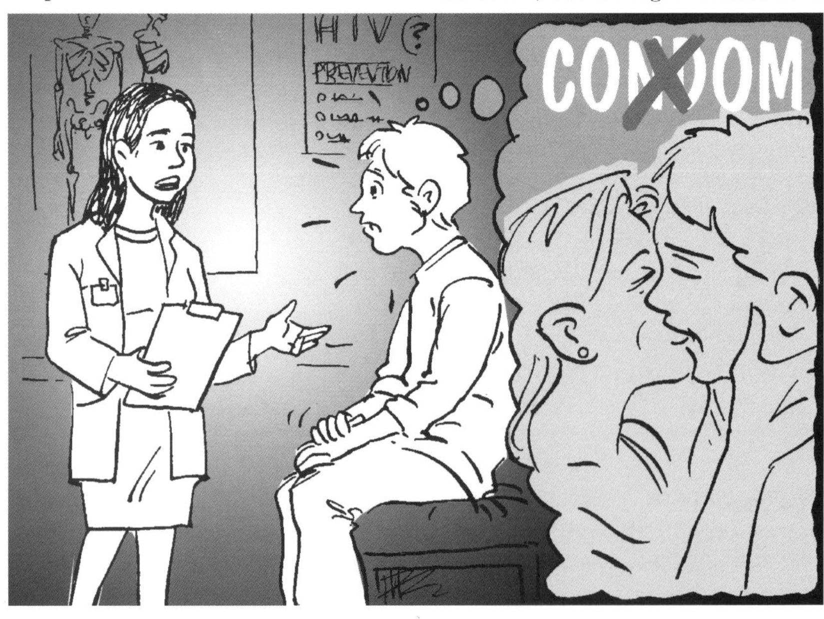

of anti-HIV drugs (combination therapy) can slow down the damaging effect of HIV on the immune system. When combination therapy is successful, it can improve the health of someone with HIV, making them less likely to develop what used to be called 'AIDS-defining conditions' and prolonging their life expectancy. In order for the anti-HIV drugs to be most effective a certain level has to be maintained in the body at all times. However, taking anti-HIV drugs can be complicated. Some people have to take a large number of pills every day with restrictions about when they have to be taken and with dietary instructions which can make it very difficult to stick to. Some of the treatments have side effects as well.

The real problems

Anti-HIV treatments have drastically improved the health of people living with HIV, but living with the virus can be stressful and difficult. Living with a potentially life-threatening infection, and knowing you could pass it on to someone else can be very difficult. Misunderstandings and fears about HIV are still widespread in society. People living with HIV may face hostility or rejection from society, some have lost jobs and homes and children have been banned from schools due to their HIV status.

If you have any concerns or questions about HIV, you can call THT Direct Helpline on 0845 1221 200 or email us at info@tht.org.uk

HIV treatments

What is combination therapy?

- It is when you take more than one type of anti-HIV treatment together.
- It works much better and for a much longer time compared to when you only take one type of anti-HIV treatment at a time (monotherapy).
- Usually combinations of three or more anti-HIV medicines are used.

What does it do?

- It prevents HIV from damaging your immune system further and allows it to recover.

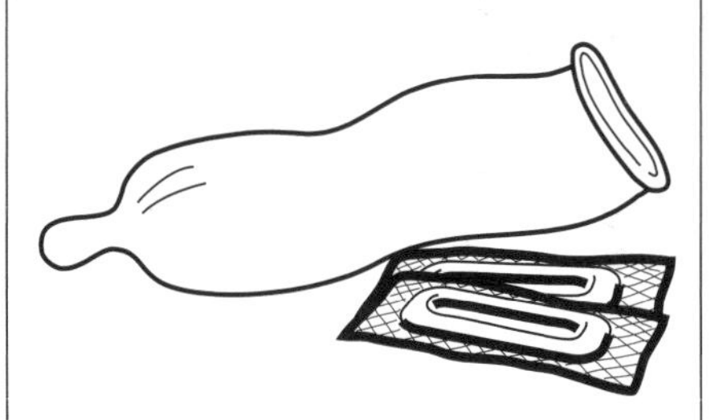

Your doctor will discuss the full details with you and you will need to go for regular check-ups to ensure all is well.

How does HIV treatment work?

HIV kills white blood cells called CD4 cells, which are important in protecting the body from infections. HIV treatment prevents HIV from multiplying and making more copies of itself in the CD4 cells. It also prevents newly produced HIV from infecting other cells in the body. Treatment limits the damage HIV does to your immune system by reducing the amount of HIV in your body. It provides your immune system with an opportunity or chance to recover from damage caused by HIV so that it starts rebuilding itself.

Most people on HIV treatment are doing well but as with all treatments and medicines, there are a few who have not done so well.

The benefits of taking combination therapy that we know of are:

- The amount of HIV in your blood will be reduced.
- Your white blood cells (CD4 count) will increase and help protect you from many infections.
- When the amount of HIV in your blood goes down, your health could improve because you are less likely to get severe infections such as tuberculosis or some types of cancer.
- The immune system strengthens over time.
- You will most likely begin to feel better.
- You are likely to live longer.
- Using three or more anti-HIV medicines from the beginning of treatment can delay the development of drug-resistant HIV.

However, we still do not know:

- What will happen if you continue using treatments for a very long time.
- How long the improvement people are experiencing will last, however many people are well five or more years after being on treatment.

We know that a small number of people are unable to tolerate the currently available anti-HIV medicines and others do not do so well.

Find out as much as possible about what taking medicines will involve, how they will make you feel and what could prevent them from working well. It will help you decide if you want to start taking them, when to start and what medicines you would consider taking. You should know:

- What the medicine does.
- How it has to be taken.
- How much to take at a time and when to take it.
- What to or what not to take it with.
- What the side effects are.
- How to store it correctly.
- How you can get someone to explain anything you do not understand about the medicine, or support you when you need help.

Ask your doctor if you do not understand anything about your treatment, no matter how simple. You could either phone or ask when you next see your doctor. Asking questions and telling your doctor what you may be worried about provides an opportunity to get help. Support groups for people taking medicines, where individuals share information with people in similar situations, run by some African organisations can be helpful. Pharmacists in the HIV clinics will discuss your treatment with you if you wish.

The information on these pages is taken from our publication *Treatment Matters*.

■ The above information is from the Terrence Higgins Trust's website which can be found at www.tht.org.uk

New HIV cases up by a fifth in a year

By Debbie Andalo

The number of new cases of HIV diagnosed in the UK has risen by 20% in one year, according to figures released 12 February 2004 by the Health Protection Agency.

There have been 5,047 new cases so far for 2003, compared with 4,204 at the same time last year. Increases in people having unsafe sex were 'undoubtedly the main driving force' behind the figures, the HPA said

Infection with HIV was increasing in both gay and heterosexual people. But the sharpest increase in new cases for 2003 was among heterosexuals – up from 2,199 to 2,785.

There were 1,414 new diagnoses among gay men in 2003, with the figure expected to rise to more than 2,000 when all reports are received. That compared with 1,195 reported early 2003 for 2002.

Dr Barry Evans, an HIV expert at the HPA, said: 'The year-on-year increase we are observing in the number of newly diagnosed HIV infections is a cause for considerable concern.

'When all reports have been received we expect the total for 2003 to be the highest ever at over 7,000. HIV is an infection that is here to stay.'

He said with almost a third of the 49,500 people currently living with HIV in the UK still unaware they are infected, the rising trend in new diagnoses is liable only to get worse before it gets better.

Some of the increase, he said, could be related to the rise in other sexually transmitted infections, which can aid the transmission of HIV, or people coming forward for HIV testing who may have been infected for some time.

But he added: 'Increases in unsafe sex are undoubtedly the main driving force behind this epidemic.'

Changing people's sexual behaviour so they use a condom with all new and casual partners was one of the most effective ways of reversing the trend, he suggested.

Nick Partridge, chief executive of Terrence Higgins Trust, said: 'We've been talking about the HIV and sexual health crisis for the last year. Now it's time for action.

There have been 5,047 new cases so far for 2003, compared with 4,204 at the same time last year

'Modernising sexual health services to make it easier for people to test for HIV and other STIs would be a major step forward in helping to tackle this crisis. We must also make a concerted and focused effort to educate young people about the risks of unprotected sex.'

The HPA recommended increased safer sex messages to the general public and reducing waiting times at clinics so people were diagnosed and treated for STIs faster.

A department of health spokesman said health promotion is crucial to reduce the spread of HIV because there is yet no cure for Aids or vaccine against HIV. He said: 'The government has made a long-term commitment through its national strategy for sexual health and HIV to improve sexual health and modernise services. HIV prevention and health promotion is a key element of this strategy.'

Testing for HIV is now offered to all first-time attendees at GUM clinics on screening for sexually transmitted infections (STIs) and to all pregnant women. But he added: 'The fact that the number of newly diagnosed cases of HIV have increased by 20% between 2002 and 2003 is truly shocking.'

Tim Yeo, shadow health and education secretary, said: 'It is time that the government listens to Conservative demands for a national service framework for sexual health and STIs. It will then be better able to set national standards and identify key interventions and ensure more is done to tackle the burgeoning public health crisis.'

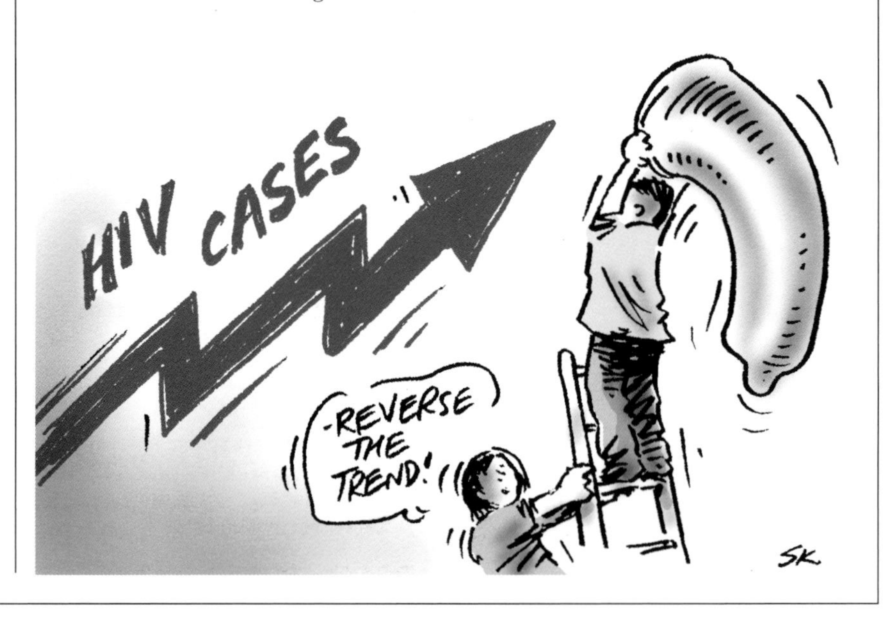

Global statistics

Information from the National AIDS Trust

AIDS kills more people worldwide than any other infectious disease and is the fourth biggest killer in Africa.

The overwhelming majority of people with HIV – some 95 per cent of the global total – live in the developing world. That proportion is set to grow even further as infection rates continue to rise in countries where poverty, conflict, poor health systems and limited resources for prevention and care fuel the spread of the virus.

More than 70 per cent of all HIV infections worldwide occur through heterosexual sex. Where this is the main form of transmission, women are becoming infected in far greater numbers than men. Women account for nearly half of all the people living with HIV and 57% in sub-Saharan Africa. Women and girls also bear the brunt of the impact of the epidemic.

Half of new infections are occurring in young people (15- to 24-year-olds), who constitute over one-quarter of those living with HIV and AIDS worldwide. Young girls are particularly at risk, with 75% of young people living with HIV in sub-Saharan Africa being women. There are an estimated 15 million children worldwide who have lost one or both parents to AIDS.

AIDS is set to reverse 50 years of development gains in the most affected countries. The economic impact of the disease can be seen in its effect on life expectancy and productivity of the workforce, tax revenues and overall loss of GDP.

UNAIDS estimates that US$20 bn will be needed by 2007 for prevention and care in low- and middle-income countries.

HIV is still a challenge in industrialised countries. Complacency over the availability of life-prolonging treatment threatens to erode safe sexual behaviour among gay men. However there remains no cure for HIV and AIDS.

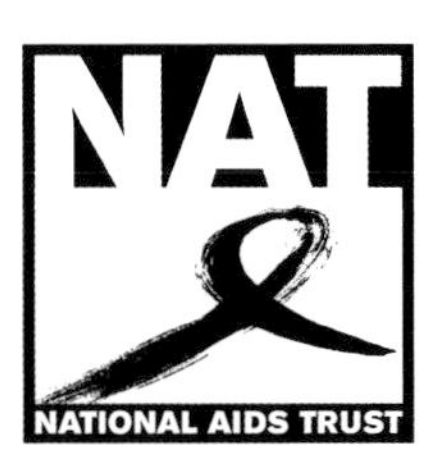

With 60% of the world's population, Asia is home to some of the fastest growing epidemics in the world with 1.1 million new infections in 2003 alone. Action is urgently needed to avoid a full-blown AIDS catastrophe in the region.

Sub-Saharan Africa

25 million people are now living with HIV and AIDS. In 2003, 3 million were newly infected with HIV.

Main mode of transmission – heterosexual sex.

Sub-Saharan Africa is by far the worst-affected region, with many countries experiencing a generalised epidemic. But there is no typical 'African' epidemic, six countries having adult prevalence rates below 2% and six above 20%.

57% of HIV-positive adults are women.

The gender difference in HIV infection is even more pronounced among 15- to 24-year-olds. The ratio ranges from 20 young women for every 10 young men in South Africa, to 45 young women for every 10 young men in Kenya.

There is a stabilisation in HIV prevalence rates but this is due to a rise in AIDS deaths and a continued increase in new infections.

Asia

7.4 million people are now living with HIV and AIDS. In 2003, 1.1 million were newly infected with HIV.

Main modes of transmission – heterosexual sex, men who have sex with men, injecting drug use.

Asia is faced with a narrow window of opportunity to prevent AIDS from having a more serious impact on the region. With 60% of the world's population, Asia is now home to some of the fastest growing epidemics in the world. This is primarily due to sharp increases in China, Indonesia and Viet Nam, which together make up close to 50% of Asia's population.

Both China and India, two of the world's most populous nations, are experiencing serious, localised epidemics.

India's national adult HIV prevalence rate of between 0.4% and

HIV and AIDS around the world

People living with HIV and AIDS	**37.8 million**
Adults	35.7 million
Women	17 million
Children under 15	2.1 million
New HIV cases in 2003	**4.8 million**
Adults	4.1 million
Children under 15	630,000
AIDS deaths in 2003	**2.9 million**
Adults	2.4 million
Children under 15	610,000
Total HIV cases to date	**57.8 million**
Total AIDS deaths to date	**20 million**

Source: National AIDS Trust

1.3% offers little indication of the serious situation facing the country. An estimated 5.1 million people were living with HIV at the end of 2003 – the second highest figure in the world, after South Africa.

In China the epidemic shows no signs of abating. Official estimates put the number of people living with HIV in China at 840,000 in 2003 but unless effective responses rapidly take hold, a total of 10 million Chinese will have acquired HIV by the end of this decade – a number equivalent to the entire population of Belgium.

In Cambodia and Thailand, national large-scale prevention programmes and political leadership have lowered HIV prevalence by up to a third. There are concerns, however, at an increase in unprotected casual sex amongst young people in Thailand and little monitoring in Cambodia of the epidemic amongst drug users and men who have sex with men.

Eastern Europe and Central Asia

1.3 million people are now living with HIV and AIDS. In 2003, 360,000 were newly infected with HIV.

Main mode of transmission – injecting drug use.

Injecting drug use is the driving force behind the epidemic. The Russian Federation has the region's worst epidemic with an estimated 3 million injecting drug users. The Ukraine has more than 600,000 injecting drug users and Kazakhstan up to 200,000.

Young people are particularly hard-hit by the epidemic with 80% of those infected under 30.

The lack of systemic surveillance in the region raises concern that HIV may be spreading amongst groups such as men who have sex with men who are not coming into contact with authorities and testing services.

Latin America and the Caribbean

2 million people are now living with HIV and AIDS. In 2003, 250,000 were newly infected.

Main modes of transmission – in South America, men who have

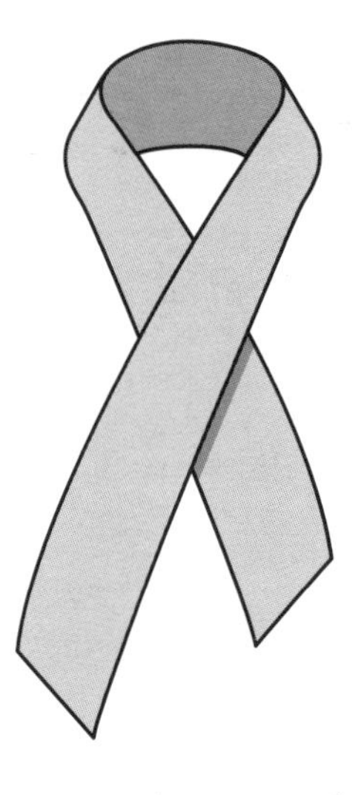

sex with men and injecting drug use; in Central America, heterosexual sex and men who have sex with men; in the Caribbean, heterosexual sex.

The Caribbean has around 430,000 people living with HIV with three countries, the Bahamas, Haiti, and Trinidad and Tobago having prevalence of over 3%.

In some South American countries such as Peru and Colombia conditions appear ripe for the virus to spread more widely as men who have unprotected sex with men also have female sexual partners.

Brazil's prevalence rates have remained stable at below 1% over the past five years, a testament to effective prevention programmes, including harm reduction and programmes amongst vulnerable groups, as well as an active and successful programme to treat HIV-positive people.

High-income countries

1.6 million people are now living with HIV and AIDS. In 2003, 64,000 were newly infected.

Main modes of transmission – heterosexual sex, men who have sex with men, injecting drug use.

Half of new infections are occurring in young people (15- to 24-year-olds), who constitute over one-quarter of those living with HIV and AIDS worldwide

Anti-retroviral drug treatments continue to reduce AIDS deaths. As a result the proportion of people living with HIV has grown.

A resurgence of sexually transmitted infection in Australia, Japan, Western Europe and the United States points to a revival of high-risk sexual behaviour, especially amongst young people and men who have sex with men. There is an obvious risk of a corresponding rise in HIV infection rates and a need to tackle complacency.

North Africa and the Middle East

480,000 people are now living with HIV and AIDS. In 2003, 75,000 were newly infected.

Main modes of transmission – heterosexual sex, injecting drug use.

Infection rates remain low although data are often unreliable.

There is little effective prevention work in the region, widespread stigmatising of vulnerable groups and little surveillance but Algeria, Lebanon and Morocco do show encouraging willingness to address the epidemic.

Countries experiencing internal and external conflicts and complex emergencies (Djibouti, Somalia, the Sudan) are particularly vulnerable to HIV epidemics. Sudan is the region's most seriously affected country with a prevalence of 2.3%.

There is concern that HIV may be spreading undetected amongst men who have sex with men as male-male sex is widely condemned and illegal in many places.

Oceania

32,000 are now living with HIV and AIDS. In 2003, 4,800 were newly infected with HIV.

Main modes of transmission – in Australia and New Zealand, men who have sex with men; in Pacific, heterosexual sex.

■ All statistics are from UNAIDS, 2004 unless otherwise indicated. Last updated: July 2004.

■ The above information is from National AIDS Trust's website which can be found at www.nat.org.uk

AIDS epidemic poses serious threat to Europe

UNAIDS and WHO call on governments to turn policy into action

With more than 1.8 million people living with HIV in Europe and Central Asia, the epidemic poses a serious threat to the region's social and economic stability, according to the Joint United Nations Programme on HIV/AIDS (UNAIDS) and the World Health Organization (WHO). UNAIDS and WHO therefore urge European governments to turn strategy into integrated HIV prevention and treatment programmes to save the lives of thousands of people.

'Countries of the newly enlarged European Union now have a prime opportunity to convert their commitment into concrete action and programmes against AIDS. Building effective partnerships is key to make a significant and sustainable contribution towards proactively addressing the HIV/AIDS epidemic in Europe,' said Dr Jack Chow, WHO's Assistant Director-General, HIV/AIDS, Tuberculosis and Malaria, ahead of the opening of a European Ministerial conference on AIDS hosted by the Government of Lithuania and the European Commission. The conference, entitled 'Europe and HIV/AIDS: New Challenges, New Opportunities', is being held from 16 to 17 September 2004 in Vilnius.

In western Europe, deaths from AIDS have declined due to the availability of HIV treatment. Alarmingly, AIDS infection rates have continued to rise because of waning government commitments to prevention efforts and complacency linked to the availability of treatment. The number of people living with HIV in western Europe rose from 540,000 in 2001 to 580,000 by end 2003.

Some of the highest infection rates in the world are in Eastern Europe, primarily in Estonia, Latvia, the Russian Federation and Ukraine where the epidemic continues to spread unchecked. HIV infections in Russia have jumped from 530,000 in 2001 to 860,000 just two years later. HIV threatens to spread relentlessly in neighbouring countries, including Belarus, Moldova, and Central Asian countries.

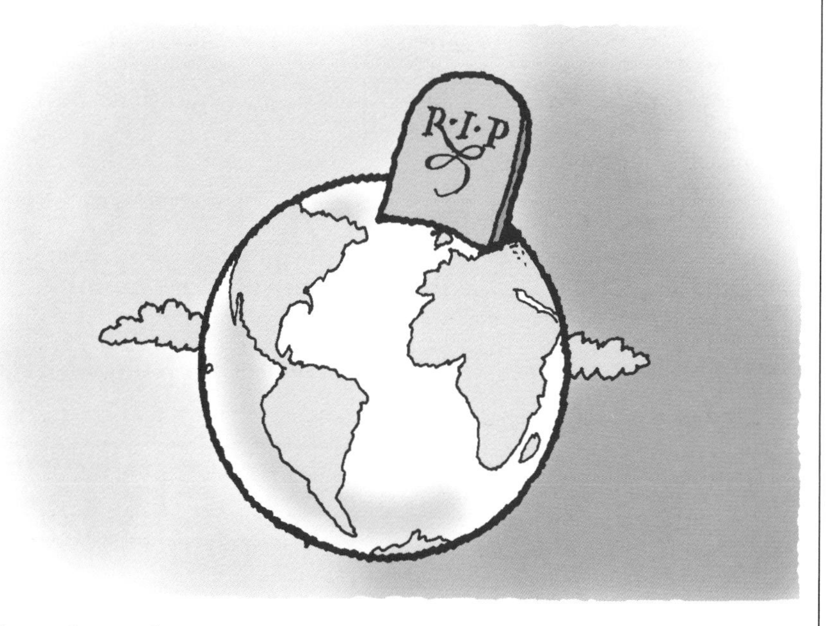

'Given that 80% of those infected in Eastern Europe are young people, there is an urgent need for a massive and comprehensive response to reduce the vulnerability of young people and empower them to become active partners in the fight against AIDS,' said Lars O. Kallings, Special Envoy of the UN Secretary-General for HIV/AIDS in Eastern Europe, who is participating in the conference. 'If no action is taken, we will be faced with a larger AIDS epidemic that risks crippling the region's social and economic development and undermining national security.'

In western Europe, deaths from AIDS have declined due to the availability of HIV treatment

Prevention is key to halting the growing AIDS epidemic. People need to be educated about the possible impact of risky behaviour and have access to condoms, needle exchange programmes and substitution therapy. Targeted awareness-raising campaigns should be carried out to inform people about how to protect themselves from HIV. As injecting drug use is the primary driver of HIV transmission in Eastern Europe, information, counselling and treatment should be made readily accessible to drug users to reduce the risk of HIV.

Countering stigma and discrimination is equally essential. Fear, ignorance, prejudice, outdated laws (including the criminalisation of drug users), and lack of information about HIV prevention and transmission all fuel the epidemic. The specific needs and challenges faced by vulnerable groups, notably drug users, sexual minorities, migrant populations, sex workers, and prisoners must be addressed comprehensively.

In Eastern Europe and Central Asia, about 15,000 people currently receive antiretroviral therapy out of 120,000 who need it. The high cost of antiretroviral (ARV) drugs is a persistent barrier to accessing antiretrovirals in Eastern Europe. Safe quality drugs must be made available to the increasing number of people who need them at affordable prices.

Cooperation among EU Member States has been critical to containing earlier waves of the epidemic. EU funding for projects led by public health experts and non-governmental organisations has enabled national actors to address the specific challenges faced by vulnerable groups. Thanks in part to Global Fund funding, countries like Albania, Moldova and Ukraine have started treatment in the past six months.

More national and European investment is urgently needed in the region. 'We would like to support the European Union for its renewed efforts to fight AIDS in Europe, particularly its commitment to assist the most-affected countries in its neighbourhood,' said Henning Mikkelsen, UNAIDS' Europe Regional Coordinator, speaking at a press conference in advance of the Ministerial conference.

■ The above information is from the World Health Organization's website which can be found at www.who.int

HIV/AIDS FAQs

Information from AVERT

AVERT
AIDS EDUCATION & RESEARCH TRUST

How many people are infected with HIV in the UK?

The Health Protection Agency (HPA) estimates that there were 49,500 adults living with HIV at the end of 2002, of whom nearly a third had not been tested and were unaware of their infection.[1]

What is the total number of HIV infections that have ever been recorded in the UK?

As of the end of June 2004, a total of 64,678 people have been diagnosed with HIV.[2]

How many people are living with AIDS in the UK? How many AIDS diagnoses have there been and how many people have died?

As of June 2004, there have been 20,501 diagnoses of AIDS in the UK. A total of 7,564 people are living with AIDS2 and 12,937 people have died of AIDS related illnesses.[3]

What age group is most affected by HIV/AIDS in the UK?

According to surveillance data produced by the HPA, people in the 25-34 age group have accounted for 45% of all HIV diagnoses in the UK.[4] However, 11% of people living with AIDS in 2001 were aged 50 or over.[5]

How many men are living with HIV compared to women?

The HPA reports a total of 28,376 (69%) men and 12,917 (31%) women living with HIV (and not AIDS) at the end of June 2004.[6] The male to female ratio of HIV diagnoses made before 1989 was more than 10 to 1, whereas in 2003 the diagnoses ratio was 5:4.[7]

Which group of people are the most affected by HIV/AIDS?

Up until the end of June 2004, it was reported that 53% of infections had occurred in men having sex with men, 38% through heterosexual sex, 7% through injecting drug use and 2% from mother to child.

Each year until 1999, there were more new HIV diagnoses in men who have sex with men than in any other group. Since then, heterosexual contact has been the major route of infection in the UK, rising to 66% of new diagnoses in 2003.[8]

As of the end of June 2004, a total of 64,678 people had been diagnosed with HIV in the UK

How many children are born with HIV in the UK?

The HPA estimates that a total of 1,151 infected children have been born to HIV infected mothers as of the end of June 2004, with a total of 225 deaths. There were 42 such births in 2002-03.[9]

Which area in the UK is most affected by HIV?

As of the end of June 2004, 58% of HIV diagnoses have been made in London.[10]

How many people are receiving drug treatments for HIV in the UK?

According to SOPHID data,[11] there were 18,448 people accessing triple or quadruple anti-retroviral therapy in England, Wales and Northern Ireland in 2002. 18,027 of these people were accessing their treatment in England.

Who are receiving drug treatments for HIV in the UK?

The British HIV Association's (BHIVA) data from their 2001-02 national audit include a breakdown of the ethnic and gender differences in those receiving treatment.[12] The audit analysed 2,044 patients from 146 centres across the UK. 73% of patients were male, 27% were female. 68% were white and 25% were black African. 44% of patients had acquired their infection heterosexually whilst 45% had acquired it gay or bisexually. 3% of infections were acquired through IV drug use.

How much does it cost to treat people with HIV in the UK?

According to the National Association of NHS Providers of AIDS Care and Treatment (PACT), the cost of managing a patient with HIV is £15,000 per year. The total cost of treatment and care in 2002-03 will be £345 million.[13] In 2000 it was estimated that the average lifetime treatment cost for an HIV-positive person was between £135,000 and £181,000.[14]

What information is collected when someone is diagnosed with HIV in the UK?

Since 2000, when someone in the UK is diagnosed as being HIV positive, a report is made to the Health Protection Agency (HPA) which includes the following data:

- If in the UK temporarily, country of usual residence
- Country of birth
- Ethnicity
- Year of arrival in the UK (if country of birth outside the UK)
- Whether the patient was presumed to be infected in the UK
- How infection was presumed to have occurred.

What information is published and where, about people who are diagnosed with HIV in the UK?

The main place where information is published is the HPA quarterly report. The HPA produce quarterly statistical tables. In addition to this a monthly report is published which sometimes contains more specific information. See www.hpa.org.uk/infections/topics_az/hiv_and_sti/hiv/epidemiology/hars.htm.

Of the HIV-positive people diagnosed in the UK who were born outside the UK, how many should be paying for their NHS treatment?

Of the 4,239 people who were born outside the UK and were diagnosed HIV positive in the UK between 2000 and 2002, it is not known how many should be paying for NHS treatment. Anyone who has been living in the UK for more than 12 months automatically qualifies for free health care. Anyone who has been in the UK for less than 12 months may qualify for free care, based on the NHS regulations.

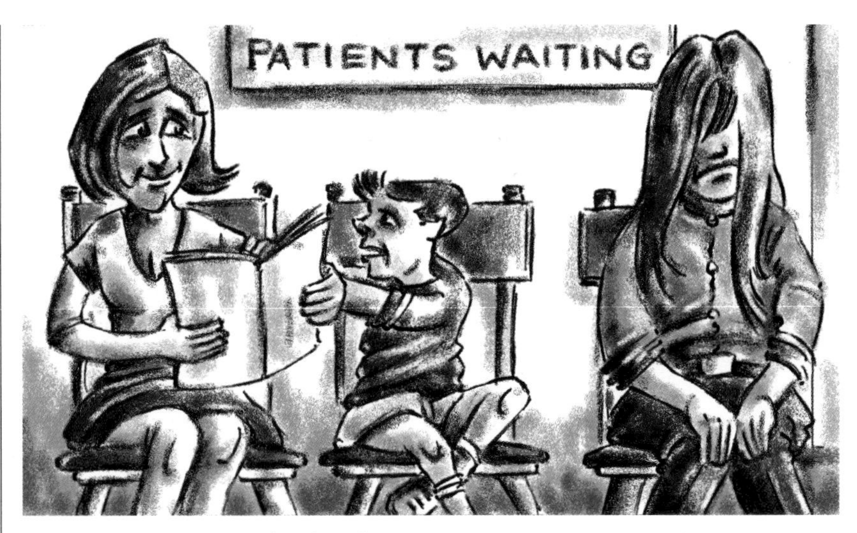

How many people diagnosed with HIV in the UK were born outside the UK?

Between 2000 and 2002, 12,312 people were diagnosed as being HIV positive. Of these, their country of birth was reported for 6,484. Of these 6,484 people, 4,239 were born outside the UK.[15]

How many people have been infected with HIV in the UK from heterosexual sex with someone who acquired the infection outside Europe in 2001 and 2002?

In 2001 and 2002, 308 people were infected with HIV from someone who had been infected outside Europe. 234 of these people were infected in Africa. This represents a rapid increase on the figures for previous years.[16]

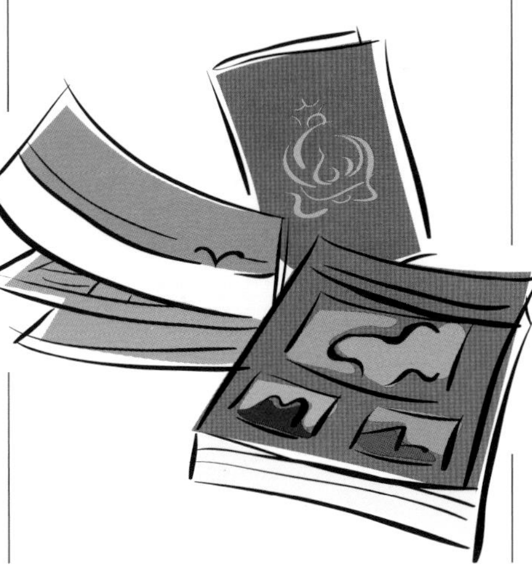

What were the countries of birth and, for those born outside the UK, the arrival dates of the people diagnosed with HIV in the UK.

This information is collected, but is not published.

Does 'health tourism' really occur?

Yes. Health tourism has always existed, as a result of inequalities between the health services of different areas and different countries. This means that people sometimes have to travel to find better or cheaper treatment. Some people may come to the UK for treatment, others may leave the UK and go elsewhere for treatment. HIV is no different from any other disease in this respect.

New guidelines are being issued by the UK government, however, to prevent treatment being given to failed asylum seekers, amongst others. The government wishes to deny help to people on the basis of their immigration status, and has set up a panel of experts to devise a plan to effect these changes.[17] Denial of treatment to many of the people in these situations, especially if they are then deported, is effectively a death sentence, and the specialists who have been asked to produce the plans have refused to do so, saying it is 'morally repugnant' and 'racist and profoundly unethical'.[18]

Ironically, the government is making efforts to supply freely the drugs to many people in their native countries who would be denied them in this country.

Don't lots of people with HIV come to the UK for treatment?

Some may. But a recent survey[20] has indicated that people living in the UK who have HIV and do not come from the UK have, on average, been living in the UK for 5 years and 1 month. More then half had been diagnosed with HIV three years ago or less. This means that most people in the UK who have HIV and do not come from the UK were unaware of their HIV status when they arrived in this country.

Are there any diseases for which people automatically get free NHS treatment, without exception?

Yes. There is a list of notifiable diseases for which anyone, regardless of their legal status, will get free NHS treatment. This is intended to prevent the spread of epidemics of infectious diseases. HIV is not on the list, but the list does include hepatitis.

What are the ethnic origins of people diagnosed as HIV positive since 2000?

Since the beginning of 2000, 16,375 diagnoses of HIV have been made in the UK. Of these ethnicity is known for 83%. Among the 13,638 whose ethnicity is known, 39% are white and 51% are black.[21]

If an HIV+ woman in the UK is pregnant, is she always guaranteed access to the drugs which will prevent her baby being born HIV+?

No. There are certain 'notifiable diseases' which are those for which a person will always receive treatment in the UK regardless of the person's legal status, in order to prevent the rapid spread of epidemics. HIV, however, is not on the notifiable diseases list. If a woman has no legal right to be in the UK – if she has overstayed a visa or is an illegal immigrant – then she will only receive medication to stop her baby being born HIV+ if doctors decide it is an 'emergency'. In some hospitals doctors will see this as an emergency, and in others they will not. Doctors are being urged to follow official guidelines, which means in some circumstances not administering drugs to prevent mother-to-child transmission of HIV.

What are the countries of origin of people diagnosed with heterosexually acquired HIV in the UK?

The data are not published. We do know the presumed countries of infection for people with heterosexually-acquired HIV diagnosed in the UK, which are shown in the table below. This does not necessarily mean that these people come from these countries – just that they were infected in them. The list includes not only high-prevalence African countries, but also popular holiday destinations.[19]

Rank	1992	1997	2002
1	Uganda	UK	Zimbabwe
2	UK	Uganda	UK
3	Zambia	Zimbabwe	S.Africa
4	Kenya	Zambia	Uganda
5	Zimbabwe	Kenya	Zambia
6	DR Congo	Nigeria	Nigeria
7	Tanzania	DR Congo	Kenya
8	Malawi	Thailand	Jamaica
9	Spain	Malawi	Malawi
10	USA	S.Africa	DR Congo

Sources:

1 Health Protection Agency, SCIEH, ISD, National Public Health Service for Wales, CDSC Northern Ireland and the UASSG. *Renewing the focus. HIV and other Sexually Transmitted Infections in the United Kingdom in 2002.* London: Health Protection Agency, November 2003.
2 HPA Communicable Disease Surveillance Centre (HIV and STI Department) and the Scottish Centre for Infection and Environmental Health: Unpublished Quarterly Surveillance Tables No. 63, 04/2, Table 1.
3 Ibid, Table 2.
4 Ibid, Table 8.
5 Age Concern England, *Opening Doors; working with older lesbians and gay men* – a resource pack, 2001.
6 HPA Communicable Disease Surveillance Centre (HIV and STI Department) and the Scottish Centre for Infection and Environmental Health: Unpublished Quarterly Surveillance Tables No. 63, 04/2, Table 1.
7 Ibid, Table 6a.
8 Ibid, Tables 6a and 6a.1.
9 Ibid, Table 14.
10 Ibid, Table 3a.
11 'Survey of Prevalent HIV Infectious Diagnosed (SOPHID) 2002'.
12 'BHIVA National Clinical Audit of ART 2001-02', Johnson, M.
13 'Sexual Health: Third Report of Session 2002-03', House of Commons Health Committee, May 2003, p. 46.
14 'The National Strategy for Sexual Health and HIV', Department of Health, 2001, p. 11.
15 HPA Behavioural Surveillance Collaborators' Meeting, 8/11/2002, Published 1/03.
16 Communicable Disease Report (CDR), AIDS and HIV infection in the United Kingdom: monthly report (July 2003). 2003;13(30).
17 *The UK Response to the HIV Epidemic: An Assessment of the UK's Compliance with the UNGASS Declaration of Commitment on HIV/AIDS*, National AIDS Trust, Aug 04.
18 *Observer* article, 8th August 2004, 'Fury at ban on HIV help for refugees'.
19 Slide presented at the Special Emphasis Surveillance Event on HIV in African Communities – held at the Communicable Disease Surveillance Centre – Health Protection Agency, 20th Feb 2004.
20 Project Nasah, Original Research Report, Feb 2003.
21 Communicable Disease Report (CDR), AIDS and HIV infection in the United Kingdom: monthly report (August 2003). 2003;13(35).

■ The above information is from AVERT's website which can be found at www.avert.org

New warning over the fast-growing HIV threat

By Sarah Boseley

The HIV virus which causes Aids and is devastating sub-Saharan Africa is now 'the fastest growing serious health condition in England', the chief medical officer said 29 July 2004.

Most people infected here have been gay men, he said in his annual report. 'However, the risk is ever present of the disease breaking through and infecting significant numbers of people in the heterosexual population in our country.'

The CMO's report points to the alarming year-on-year rise in the numbers of people becoming infected and the failure of clinics to cope with the need to test those at risk. People who do not know they are HIV positive will fuel the epidemic by infecting new sexual partners.

Between 1996 and 1997, new infections rose by just 42, from 2,479 to 2,521. But since 2000, the numbers have increased by a little under 1,000 a year.

The last year for which there are complete figures is 2002, when 5,615 people became infected. The estimate for 2003 is more than 7,000 – the highest ever. The fastest growth is in people infected through heterosexual sex in Africa, but infections from heterosexual sex outside of Africa are also rising.

At the end of 2002, an estimated 43,500 people in England were carrying the HIV virus, but a third of them did not know it, the report said. The CMO, Sir Liam Donaldson, highlighted HIV as a major concern because of inadequate testing for the virus, which means that people ignorant of their HIV status may infect others and that some people with the virus may die because their condition is not identified in time.

People who do not know they are HIV positive will fuel the epidemic by infecting new sexual partners

Opportunities to test those at highest risk are not being taken, the report said. About 59% of men who have sex with men and visit a genito-urinary medicine clinic leave with their HIV status undiagnosed.

Every pregnant woman should be offered a test, because treatment can prevent transmission of the infection to the baby. But in London a quarter of HIV-positive pregnant women are not tested, and 13% are not tested in the rest of England.

This lack of testing 'has serious implications for the HIV/Aids epidemic in England. Urgent improvements need to be made,' said the report.

People are having to wait up to six weeks to have a sexually transmitted infection diagnosed, health campaigners said at the launch of a report by the Health Protection Agency on the soaring rate of other infections.

Early results of a pilot study by the HPA into waiting times at GUM clinics are worrying, said the CMO's report. More than a quarter – 28% – of emergencies were not seen within 48 hours and 8% waited longer than two weeks. Only 18% of people making routine appointments were seen within 48 hours and 41% were waiting for over two weeks.

'This report and the figures released on sexually transmitted infections underline the appalling state of the UK's sexual health,' said Nick Partridge, chief executive of the Terrence Higgins Trust. He called for more investment in services.

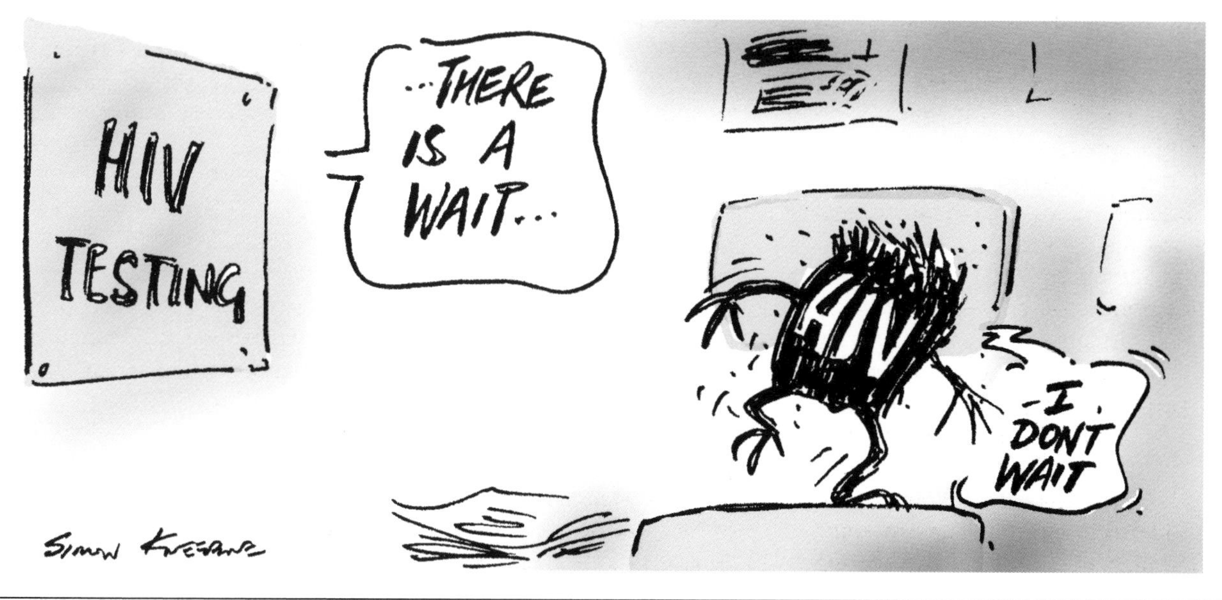

HIV/AIDS and adolescents

Information from the United Nations Population Fund (UNFPA)

HIV/AIDS has become a disease of young people, with young adults aged 15-24 accounting for half of the some 5 million new cases of HIV infection worldwide each year. Yet young people often lack the information, skills and services they need to protect themselves from HIV infection. Providing these is crucial to turning back the epidemic.

An estimated 6,000 youth a day become infected with HIV/AIDS – one every 14 seconds – the majority of them young women. At the end of 2001, an estimated 11.8 million young people aged 15-24 were living with HIV/AIDS, one-third of the global total of people living with HIV/AIDS. Only a small percentage of these young people know they are HIV-positive.

In addition, more than 13 million children under age 15 have lost one or both parents to AIDS. The overwhelming majority of these AIDS orphans live in Africa. By 2010, their number is projected to reach 25 million.

Contributing factors

A combination of social, biological and economic factors helps fuel the AIDS pandemic:

Poverty

HIV/AIDS is a disease highly associated with poverty. A World Bank study of 72 countries showed that both low per capita income and high-income inequality were linked to high national HIV infection rates, and a $2,000 increase in per capita income was associated with a 4 per cent reduction in infections. The 2001 United Nations General Assembly Special Session on HIV/AIDS recognised that 'poverty, underdevelopment and illiteracy are among the principal contributing factors to the spread of HIV/AIDS'.

Girls and women are more vulnerable

For reasons of biology, gender and

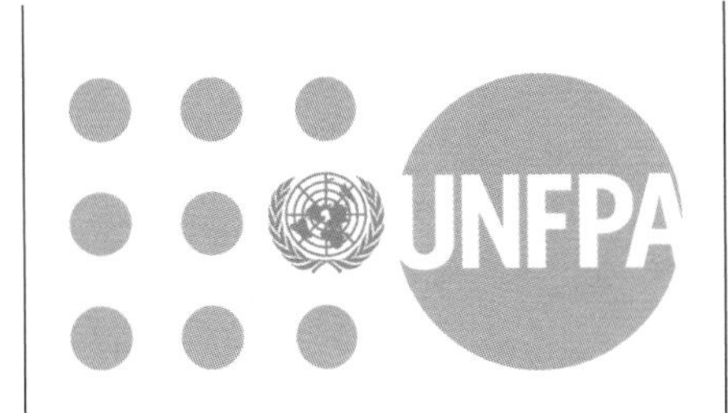

cultural norms, females are more susceptible than males to HIV infection. Thus an estimated 7.3 million young women are living with HIV/AIDS compared to 4.5 million young men. Two-thirds of newly infected youth aged 15-19 in sub-Saharan Africa are female. Among women, the peak age for HIV prevalence tends to be around age 25, 10 to 15 years younger than the peak age for men.

Biologically, the risk of infection during unprotected sex is two to four times higher for women than men; young women are even more vulnerable because their reproductive tracts are still maturing and tears in the tissue allow easy access to infection.

Socially, young women also face higher risks. When they have sexual relations, it tends to be with older men, increasing the likelihood that their partners are already infected. Some adolescent girls are attached to 'sugar daddies', much older, relatively well-off (usually married) men who support them in exchange for sex. More commonly, sexually active adolescent girls, in Africa at least, have partners 2-10 years their senior who provide them with gifts, such as soap, perfume, meals out and jewellery. Some poor girls exchange sex for money for school fees or to help their families. Once in these relationships with teachers, drivers, shopkeepers or even policemen, girls have little power to negotiate the use of condoms.

Men often seek younger sexual partners who are unlikely to be infected with HIV.

The common myth in some places that sex with a virgin can cure AIDS or STIs further endangers young girls who fall prey to forced or coerced sexual relations.

Married youth at risk

Marriage does not always protect young women against HIV infection. Since a much higher percentage of young men than young women become sexually active early, young women are likely to marry an already sexually experienced man. In Pune, India, a study in an STI clinic found that 25 per cent of the 4,000 women attending the clinic were

Young people and HIV/AIDS

Young people aged 15-24 living with HIV/AIDS, by sex, December 2001

Region	Young women	Young men	Total
Sub-Saharan Africa	67%	33%	8,600,000
North Africa and the Middle East	41%	59%	160,000
East Asia and the Pacific	49%	51%	740,000
South Asia	62%	38%	1,100,000
Central Asia and Eastern Europe	35%	65%	430,000
Latin America and the Caribbean	31%	69%	560,000
Industrialised countries	33%	67%	240,000
World	62%	38%	11,800,000

Source: UNICEF/UNAIDS/WHO

infected with an STI and 14 per cent were HIV-positive. Among the 93 per cent who were married, 91 per cent had only one partner, their husbands.

A study in Kisumu, Kenya, found that as many as half of the married women whose husbands were 10 or more years older were infected with HIV, compared to none of the women whose husbands were only up to three years older.

Within marriage it is particularly difficult for women to negotiate condom use, especially if they are much younger than their husbands.

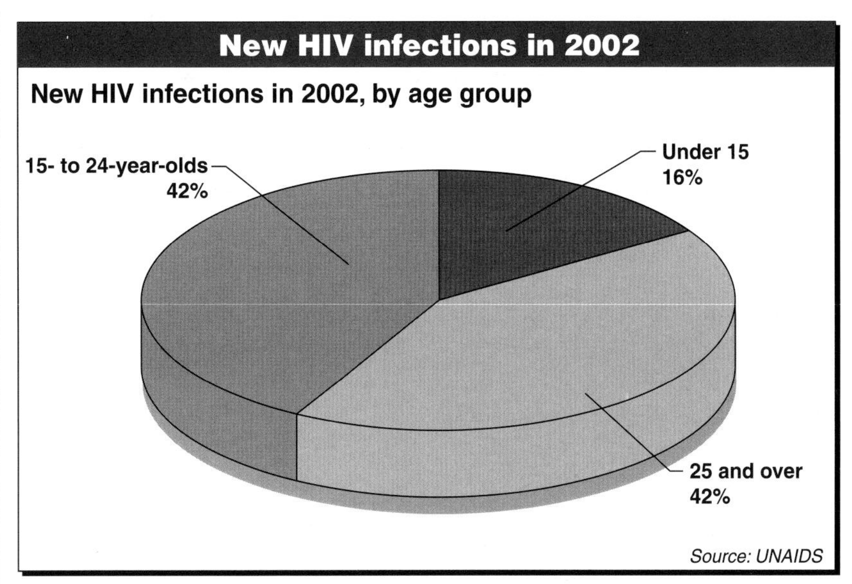

Lack of information and skills for protection

Because sex is a taboo topic in many countries, large numbers of young people do not get sufficient information – or the skills – to refuse sex or negotiate safer sex practices. While most young people have heard about HIV/AIDS, few know enough to protect themselves against infection.

Surveys from 40 countries indicate that more than half of the young people have misconceptions about how HIV is transmitted. In Ukraine, while 100 per cent of adolescent females know about AIDS, only 21 per cent know of three methods of prevention. In Somalia, only 26 per cent of adolescent females have heard of AIDS and only 1 per cent know how to protect themselves. In Botswana, where one in three people is living with HIV/AIDS, virtually all young people have heard of AIDS and more than 75 per cent know the three primary means of protection. Still, 62 per cent of girls had at least one major misconception about how HIV is spread. Far too many young people think they can tell if someone is HIV-positive simply by looking at them.

Feelings of invincibility

Adolescents tend to underestimate, downplay or deny their risks of HIV infection. Case studies by the World Health Organization (WHO) indicate that only between one-fifth and one-third consider themselves at risk. Many young people do not recognise that their partner's behaviour also puts them at risk. Still others may perceive HIV as something that occurs only among sex workers, drug users or men who share intimate relations. Feelings of invincibility, combined with the lack of awareness of the consequences of risky behaviour, may make them less likely to take precautions to protect their health – and lives.

Sexually transmitted infections

Sexually transmitted infections increase the likelihood of HIV transmission considerably, as well as having other reproductive health consequences such as chronic pain, infertility or life-threatening ectopic pregnancies. While data on STIs in developing countries are scarce, particularly for young people, WHO estimates that at least a third of the more than 333 million new cases of curable STIs each year occur among people under age 25. Young people are also substantially more likely than adults to become re-infected after having been treated.

> ***Young people are more likely to seek traditional remedies for STIs, or to ignore the symptoms. This pattern is attributed to feelings of guilt over having an STI***

A study in South Africa showed that adolescent girls were 30 per cent more likely to get STIs than were boys, in large part because they were involved with older males who were more likely to have STIs themselves.

Studies on gonorrhoea in selected Middle Eastern and African countries found infection levels were highest among the 15-19 age group. A substantial minority of young people, more men than women, have experienced symptoms of STIs, according to studies from Argentina, Botswana, Peru, the Philippines, the Republic of Korea and Thailand.

Knowledge about STIs is generally poor among young people. A study among young sex workers in Cambodia found that their limited knowledge was based on a mixture of facts, myths and rumours and was not always correct. An unfortunate misconception among many young people, including in Kampala, Uganda, and Ho Chi Minh City, Viet Nam, is that STI symptoms will go away over time or that good personal hygiene will prevent STIs (and HIV). One in five female university students in Ilorin, Nigeria, 30 per cent of youth in parts of Chile and half of young men and women in sites in Guatemala also hold this belief.

Young people are more likely to seek traditional remedies for STIs, or to ignore the symptoms. This pattern is attributed to feelings of guilt over having an STI and to the stigmatising treatment they tend to receive in health care centres, including STI clinics.

Alcohol and drug use

Sharing needles for drug use is a highly efficient means of spreading HIV because the virus is injected directly into the blood stream. Mixing drug use with sex for money provides a bridge for HIV from injecting drug users to the wider community.

Drug use often starts in adolescence. In Nepal, where half of the country's 50,000 injecting drug users are 16 to 25 years old, the incidence of HIV among people who inject drugs climbed from 2 per cent in 1995 to nearly 50 per cent in 1998. The Russian Federation's HIV epidemic is the fastest growing in the world, fuelled by the rising number of young drug users. In China, HIV rates are highest among injecting drug users, typically young men.

The number of drug addicts is rising, particularly in Eastern and Central Europe, as is the number of occasional users. According to 2000 figures from UNAIDS, injecting drug use accounts for more than half of all HIV cases in Argentina, Bahrain, China, Georgia, Iran, Italy, Kazakhstan, Latvia, Moldova, Portugal, the Russian Federation, Spain and Ukraine.

Alcohol use can also fuel the HIV epidemic by increasing risky sexual behaviour. A study in Rwanda found that young people aged 15-24 who consumed alcohol were less likely to abstain from sex. In a study of young adolescents in Jamaica, those who had experimented with alcohol were 2.4 times more likely than others to say they had sexual activity, other factors being equal.

Interaction with tuberculosis

Tuberculosis is the leading cause of death among AIDS patients worldwide. One-third of all AIDS patients are infected with tuberculosis. Those infected with HIV are much more likely than others – 800 times, by some estimates – to develop active tuberculosis. In Kenya, the prevalence of both HIV and tuberculosis doubled between 1990 and 1996.

Young people should receive vaccinations to prevent tuberculosis. Most tuberculosis is treatable using directly observed therapy. Leaving it half-treated or mistreated can result in drug-resistant tuberculosis, which is harder and much more expensive to treat. Thus, tuberculosis control programmes, including for young people, must be an integral part of AIDS prevention and care strategies.

Sharing needles for drug use is a highly efficient means of spreading HIV because the virus is injected directly into the blood stream

Impact of AIDS on young people

Adolescent orphans

Youth who have lost one or both parents to AIDS are particularly vulnerable to infection themselves. Many face exploitation, including physical and sexual abuse. With weakened family support, some engage in risky sexual behaviour or inject drugs. Those forced to live on the streets may turn to sex work and crime as a means to survive. After suffering the emotional toll of losing their parents, many also face stigma and discrimination.

Education

Young people infected or affected by HIV/AIDS frequently have their schooling disrupted. Dropping out is common, particularly for girls who have to care for sick family members or their siblings to keep the family together. Inability to pay school fees also forces boys and girls to leave school. Others drop out because of stigma and discrimination by schools, teachers or classmates.

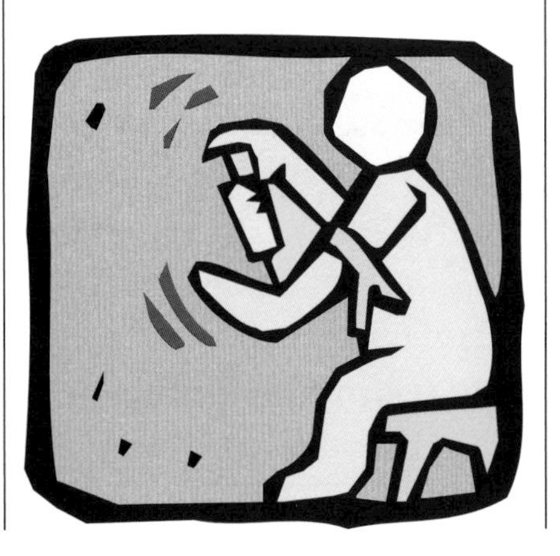

Teachers are also succumbing to HIV/AIDS. UNAIDS estimates that in 2001 as many as 1 million children and young people in sub-Saharan Africa lost their teachers to AIDS.

Growing up without an education has lifetime effects. Survey data from countries around the world show that when parents are not alive, children aged 10-14 are less likely to be in school than are children of the same age whose parents are alive. In Madagascar, for example, the percentage of orphaned children aged 10-14 in school is 34 per cent compared to 65 per cent of non-orphaned children. In Indonesia, the percentages are 65 and 85, respectively.

The ABC approach

In 2001, the United Nations General Assembly Special Session (UNGASS) endorsed the ABC approach to preventing HIV infection. The ABC approach to behaviour change gives three clear messages for preventing the transmission of HIV. ABC stands for: Abstain from having sexual relations or, for youth, delay having sex; Be faithful to one uninfected partner; and use Condoms consistently and correctly.

Sometimes D, for Drugs, is added to the message, referring to intravenous drug use and recreational use of alcohol, which can increase the likelihood of unsafe sex. Some also refer to ABC+, which includes the message to get tested and treated for STIs (which increase the risk of transmission of HIV in unprotected sex). Each component of the ABC message should be presented in a comprehensive and balanced way.

■ The above information is an excerpt of chapter three, HIV/AIDS and Adolescents, of the *State Of World Population 2003* report produced by the United Nations Population Fund. For a full list of references see http://www.unfpa.org/swp/2003/english/sources.htm

Carry on up the campus

Student life can be fraught with one-night stands and seventies revival nights, but what do our bright young things care about sex bugs and the global fight for cheap Aids drugs? Rebecca Holman finds out

Freshers' is the perfect opportunity for many young people leaving home for the first time to week drink far too much, experiment with drugs and have casual sex. For some, the fun doesn't stop with the first week of term. With different parties and events organised throughout the year it is easy to look back on your time at university as one long haze of cider-infused cocktails, seventies revival nights and ill-advised one night-stands with geography students.

As fun as all this sounds, one of the consequences is a worrying rise in the number of sexually-transmitted infections among young people, with 1.5 million attendances reported at GUM clinics in England, Wales and Northern Ireland during 2002. This translates to a 15 per cent increase on the previous year.

This increase is largely made up of a huge increase in STI diagnoses among young people. Ten times as many young women aged 16-24 were diagnosed with chlamydia in 2000/1 than any other age group; three times as many as young men.

Chlamydia may currently be the most common STI in the UK, but it is by no means the only one affecting students. Levels of gonorrhoea and syphilis have increased sharply in the past decade or so too, with young people bearing the brunt of the increase and, particularly with the last two infections, young gay men.

Sexually-transmitted infections are, of course, no big secret for young people, and most universities run some sort of sexual health awareness campaign.

More awareness needed on campus

Students and young people can be particularly lax when it comes to practising safer sex, with the fear of unwanted pregnancies often being seen as the only issue worth worrying about.

Hannah Briggs, a 20 year-old student from Leeds, admits that although sexual health promotions exist in universities, they do not raise much awareness among students. 'The messages tend to go in one ear and out the other.'

She explains: 'Most universities are good for trying to promote awareness, but students just don't know how easy it is to catch things or how widespread they are.' Hannah warns that girls should be especially careful as, in her experience, young men will never bother to get tested, and are 'totally clueless'. In fact she may be right here. On a global level and according to SPW (Student Partnerships Worldwide), teenage girls and women are nearly five to seven times more likely to contract HIV than their (straight) male counterparts.

Denise is Nurse Manager at the medical centre of King's College, London. She feels that much of the problem lies with sexual health clinics becoming inundated, particularly in the capital. This leaves long waiting times at the drop-in services and difficulty in making appointments.

An alternative is to offer the same services as GUM clinics at university medical centres. But there is no standardisation here. Some clinics offer a full range of services while others only provide a nurse drop-in service.

King's College, London offers a wide, though by no means complete range of services (but they do more than most GPs). Denise admits: 'One of the problems lies in the attitudes of the students, who are aware it's a problem, but for other people.' This is despite colleges like King's putting on their own sexual health awareness events, many of which coincide once a year with World Aids Day. In King's case this is SHAG: Sexual Health And Guidance.

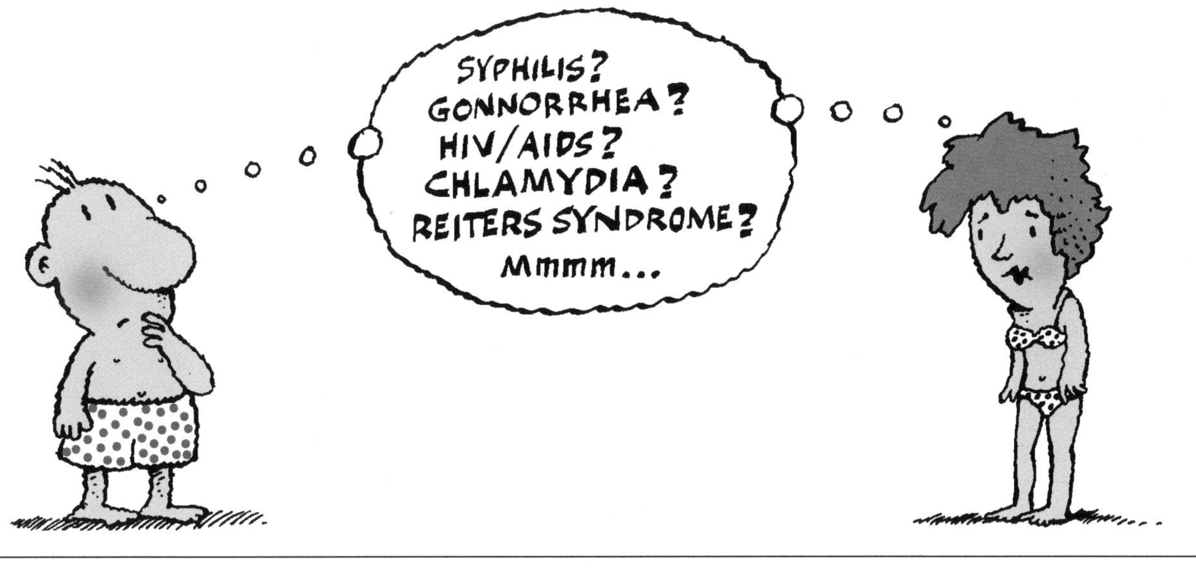

Even when it does affect them, Denise says, 'they don't necessarily do something about it.'

Clearly it's not just the services available that have to change, but the attitudes of those who use them.

The Student Stop Aids Campaign university tour

SPW (Student Partnerships Worldwide) took matters of student apathy into its own hands when it launched the Students Stop Aids Campaign (SSAC) earlier this year. They set up Students Stop Aids societies at Freshers' Fairs across the country. Six youth organisations now support the campaign.

An SSAC speakers' tour of 11 universities took place at the end of October in which several young people from around the world discussed the ways in which HIV and Aids have affected their lives with some of the students from the universities involved.

According to Jenny Ross, campaigns and advocacy manager for the SSAC, the aim of the tour was to 'raise awareness on campuses of the global Aids epidemic,' though this was to be done in a fairly informal manner, not as a lecture with an academic format.

Jenny says: 'Young people are the group most affected by HIV and Aids globally, and are also the group with the best chance of tackling this epidemic. This is why students have come together in this campaign to make demands.'

The tour enabled speakers to share their experiences of the Aids epidemic with young people in the UK. It was officially launched with a parliamentary debate.

Jenny has been impressed by the response young people across the country have given the tour, estimating that it reached 1,700 people directly, and many more through interviews given on local BBC and commercial radio.

She was struck by one thing, however, that: 'Young people have no sense of what it is like to be HIV positive.'

She hopes that the tour will make young people more aware of their sexual behaviour, and feels that it is important for young people to mobilise themselves: 'this is a crisis of our generation. Older people and those in authority are reluctant to recognise young people are having sex, and healthcare professionals need to be more aware of how they talk to young people.'

Uganda's Sentuma Sparks, a 24-year-old IT student, was one of the speakers on the SSAC tour. He became interested in Aids prevention work when he saw how poverty and lack of empowerment among young people allowed the Aids crisis to flourish in his own country. 'There is much more information on sexual health awareness available to young people in the UK,' says Sparks. 'But they don't necessarily know where to look for it. And they sometimes lack the political will that can be found in Ugandans.'

'Young people are the group most affected by HIV and Aids globally, and are also the group with the best chance of tackling this epidemic'

Clint Walters, 24, runs the UK's HIV peer support group HIFY (Health Initiatives for Young People with HIV), and also took part on the SSAC tour. He praised it as 'a good stepping stone' for future work with young people. However, he was shocked too to discover that most students attending had very little in-depth knowledge of HIV and Aids, thus emphasising the need to generate awareness among young people. Clint was also surprised to learn that he was the only HIV positive speaker on the tour, indicating how difficult young positive people find it to speak out.

There is no standardised compulsory sex education on the national curriculum in the UK, and this could go along way to explain why such stigma and lack of awareness exists. 'It is still a huge uphill battle,' continues Clint, 'but the success of the Student Stop Aids university speaker tour, and the interest generated by it, are certainly positive signs.'

Students make good advocates and campaigners

It is not just issues of sexual health awareness in the UK that the speaker tour raised. Awareness of the global Aids crisis was also a prevalent theme.

Jenny Ross believes that young people are not as apathetic as we are sometimes led to believe. 'The war in Iraq showed that young people are interested in international issues, not apathetic and selfish'.

SPW organises programmes where volunteers (often students taking a year out) can travel to countries in Africa and Asia and live among communities working as peer educators in rural primary and secondary schools for between seven to nine months. Many of these students, on their return to the UK, have become cornerstones of their Students Stop Aids Societies, putting the invaluable skills they learnt abroad to good use here.

So maybe students aren't all as lazy, selfish and apathetic as some of the evidence suggests. However, we still have to ask, if students across the country can get so fired up about the war in Iraq, why can't they get fired up over the global Aids crisis, which is causing the death and suffering of many more people? Why can't they get fired up enough to worry about their own sexual health and that of their peers?

What is currently missing from young people is the political will and motivation to look at the issues being raised, and it is here that SPW seems to have the right idea. However there is still a long way to go before young people in the UK are managing their sexual health in the way they should. Until then, just remember to avoid cider – and dodgy 70s nights!

■ To get more involved in student activities, visit the websites www.stopaidscampaign.org.uk and www.spw.com HIFY – HIV peer support for young people: Tel Freefone 0800 298 3099.

■ The above information is from *Positive Nation*, the magazine published by the UKC – the UK Coalition of People Living with HIV and AIDS. Visit the website at www.positivenation.co.uk

HIV/AIDS now a disease of young people . . .

. . . especially girls and women

HIV/AIDS has become a disease of young people, with half of all new infections occurring in 15- to 24-year-olds, according to UNFPA's *The State of World Population 2003* report. An estimated 6,000 youth become infected with HIV/AIDS each day – one every 14 seconds – the majority of them young women.

The fastest spread of HIV/AIDS among youth is in sub-Saharan Africa, where an estimated 8.6 million youth (67 per cent female) are infected, followed by South Asia where some 1.1 million youth are infected (62 per cent female).

Discussing sexual behaviour is taboo in many countries and information activities are inadequate, so large numbers of young people do not have the information or skills to refuse sex or negotiate safer sexual practices, says the report, *Making 1 Billion Count: Investing in Adolescents' Health and Rights*. In Somalia, only 26 per cent of adolescent females have heard of AIDS and only 1 per cent know how to protect themselves.

Poverty is also a major factor for HIV infection. Some poor girls exchange sex for money for school fees or to help their families, placing them at risk of infection. The report also indicates that married adolescent girls are at particular risk since they are often married to older men with more sexual experience and are generally unable to negotiate condom use. Recent research in Kenya and Zambia suggests that married girls are more likely to be HIV positive than their unmarried counterparts.

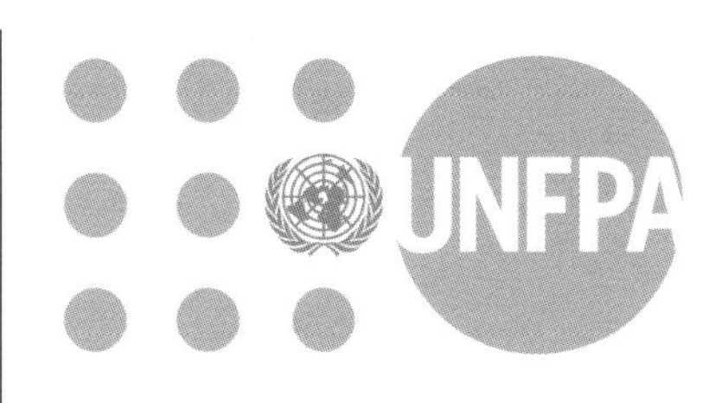

The provision of accurate, age-appropriate information and services for youth is crucial, stresses the report. Teaching the 'ABC' approach, Abstinence, Be faithful, and use Condoms has proven effective, especially in Africa. The 'Million Voices' initiative in South Africa, for example, aims to reach 3 million young people with sexuality education through youth centres within three years. Nevertheless, negative perceptions about condom use persist. In a study in Kenya, only 35 per cent of urban students and 56 per cent of rural students expressed confidence in the effectiveness of condoms.

Youth-friendly voluntary counselling and testing services (VCT) are vital since only a small percentage of young people with HIV realise they are infected. Regardless of the result, the report argues, young people tend to take fewer risks after being tested. In a study in Kenya and Uganda, VCT was offered to young people aged 14 to 21 and most sought the test when they were healthy. In interviews after being tested, most said they intended to abstain, keep to one partner, have fewer partners or use condoms.

■ UNFPA's *State of World Population* report has been published annually since 1978. Chapter 3 of the 2003 report focuses on the impact of HIV/AIDS on adolescents. The full report is available online at www.unfpa.org

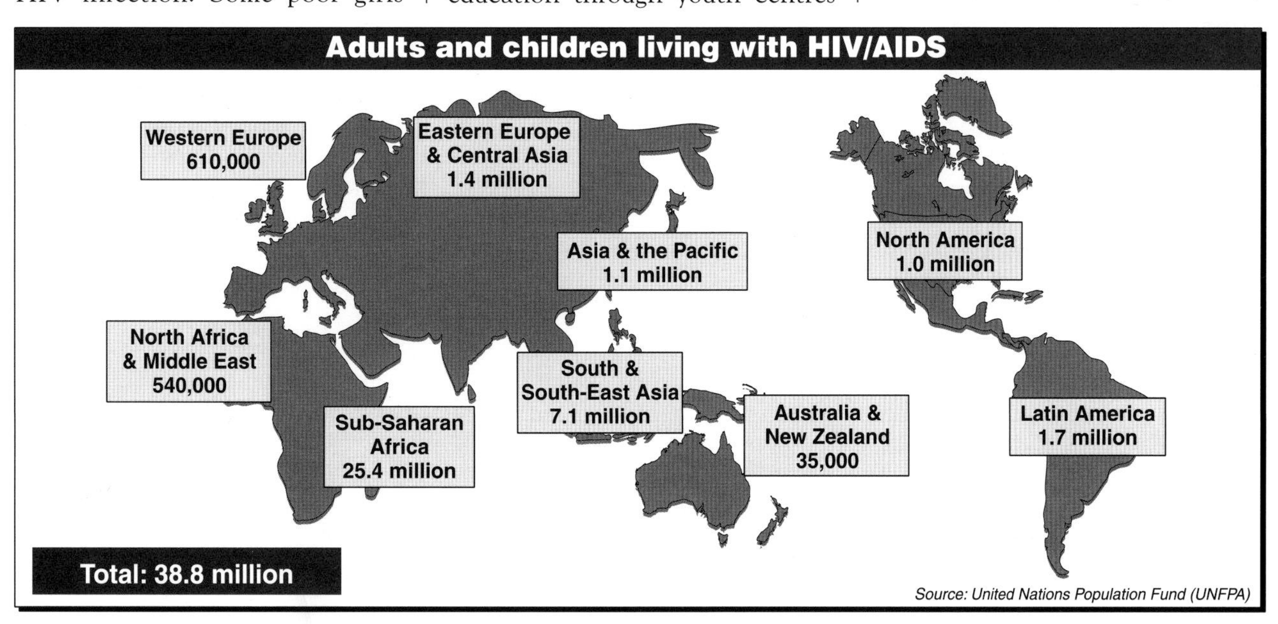

Record numbers infected

Aids defeating world's best efforts as record numbers are infected

By Sarah Boseley, Health Editor

The lethal spread of the HIV/Aids pandemic across the globe is speeding up, in spite of intensifying efforts on the part of UN agencies, the US, Britain and other European governments to turn the tide. A record five million people were infected by the virus last year and nearly three million died.

The UN's latest bi-annual report on the state of the pandemic made it plain 6 July 2004 that the HIV virus that causes Aids is defeating man's best efforts to contain it. There are 38 million people carrying the virus, sub-Saharan Africa is being devastated, and the fastest spread is in Asia and eastern Europe.

'More people than in any previous year became infected with HIV. That is clearly a failure to reach the people who need it with prevention methods. More people than ever before died of Aids. That is a failure to reach them with treatment,' said Peter Piot, executive director of Unaids, at the launch of the report in London 6 July 2004. The epidemic, he said, is reaching its global phase, and is no longer a problem largely confined to sub-Saharan Africa.

One in every four new infections is occurring in Asia, where huge populations are at risk, said the report, published just before the international Aids conference in Bangkok, July 2004. There have been sharp increases in the numbers infected in China, Indonesia and Vietnam, while India alone has 5.1 million people with HIV – the second largest number infected in any country, after South Africa.

In eastern Europe and central Asia, 1.3 million have the virus, spread largely by injecting drug use. Russia, with more than three million injecting drug users and 860,000 with HIV, is one of the worst hit.

It is a dispiriting picture, because more work and money is going into the battle against the world's worst disease outbreak than ever before, both in helping people to protect themselves against contracting the virus and more recently in efforts to get drugs that can prevent HIV developing into Aids to people in poor countries.

But still not enough is being done, said Dr Piot. 'The world is falling short on prevention. Preventing new infections will at the end of the day stop this epidemic,' he said. 'Only one in five who need it have access to HIV prevention – [such as] education of children in schools, access to condoms and access to clean needles for those who are injecting drugs.'

Limited progress

There had been some progress on treatment, he said, but too little. There are now about 440,000 people in the developing world on Aids drugs, which keep the level of the virus in the blood low, although they are not a cure. Half of those people are in Brazil, although the drugs are becoming more available in Asia. Where they are most needed – in sub-Saharan Africa with its 25 million infected and where 2.2 million people died of Aids last year – the antiretroviral drugs that can keep people alive are still rare. Treatment, said Dr Piot, 'is still dramatically, shockingly low in Africa'.

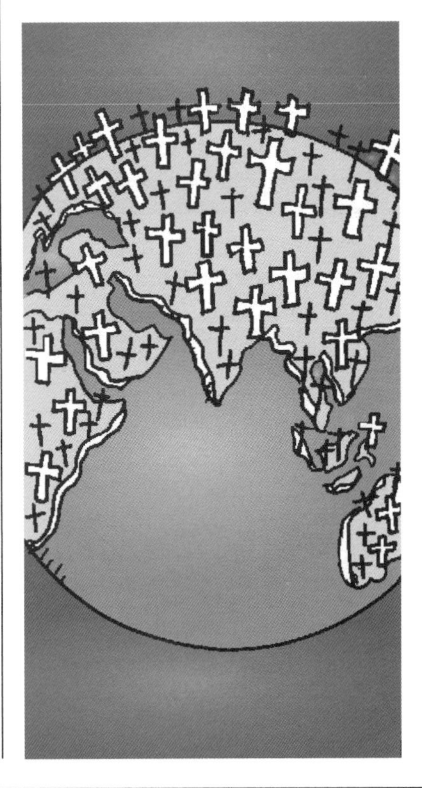

He expects it to improve. The World Health Organisation has set a target of three million people on treatment by 2005 and international funds are being made available to poor countries that want to put into place treatment plans. President George Bush has pledged $15bn (£8.1bn) over five years to fight Aids, which the US has recognised as a threat to world security. Philanthropic foundations, such as that of Bill and Melinda Gates and also Bill Clinton, are putting money and muscle into the struggle.

But nobody was underestimating the scale of the challenge, even though drug prices have come down dramatically.

Many of the worst-affected countries are hard-pressed to draw up treatment plans and are very short of nurses, doctors and hospitals, even without the Aids epidemic. They need to train people to administer the drugs and overcome the stigma of the disease to persuade people to come forward for testing before they become sick.

But there is little alternative. Prevention efforts have been successful in a few countries such as Thailand and Uganda but have not slowed the pandemic and need a rethink, said Dr Piot.

For many women in Africa, the mantra of ABC – abstinence, be faithful and condoms – which is regularly recited by outside agencies and especially the US is 'pretty irrelevant', he said.

The Aids pandemic in Africa is hitting women worst. Nearly 60% of the victims are female, and they often do not have the option of abstinence, fidelity or condom use. Many are subject to violent, non-consensual sex by men.

'To ensure women become less infected, we have to target men,' said Dr Piot. 'We are getting into a need for quite fundamental and long-ranging behaviour change. We have to change norms in society.'

One of the best hopes for women, he said, was the development of a microbicide – a drug that can prevent the transmission of HIV during intercourse.

Clare Short, as international development secretary, put substantial British funding into microbicide research, which has not yet borne fruit, although her successor, Hilary Benn, said 6 July 2004 that five clinical field trials were about to get under way.

The UK is the second biggest donor to HIV/Aids initiatives, and on 6 July 2004 Mr Benn announced a further £116m to two UN agencies involved in the fight – Unaids and the United Nations Population Fund. He also launched a paper setting out how the Department for International Development plans to push for high quality family planning in developing countries.

'Sexual and reproductive health and Aids are inextricably linked. By taking action on one, we know we are also helping to tackle the other,' he said.

The statistics in the Unaids report have been collated from a number of sources, including countries' own estimates of the numbers infected, surveys and data from anonymous testing of women at antenatal clinics.

Unaids says some of the estimates are lower than previously, because of improved methodology, but there is no doubt of the upward trend of infections and deaths.

AIDS pandemic out of control in many nations

Information from Aids Care, Education and Training (ACET)

By Dr Patrick Dixon

More than 85 million people have become infected already with the virus causing AIDS. In many countries the spread of HIV is out of control. We are in a race against time. Many communities in Africa have been devastated yet the greatest impact is still to come from an illness which can take more than a decade to develop. We are seeing rapid spread now in India, Russia, China and many other places.

It is hard for many people in Western countries to imagine what it is like knowing that maybe a third of all parents of school children in your city are going to die soon of AIDS, a third of your office team, a third of your church congregation even – people may find faith and join a church but they will continue to be infected, barring a miracle.

The AIDS crisis has deepened despite efforts over the last 15 years. We need national programmes in hard-hit areas on a scale never seen before, encouraged by success in containing spread where government, media, community and churches, as well as other faith-based organisations, have worked together.

AIDS can be beaten but need to act now

AIDS is caused by the human immunodeficiency virus, HIV. HIV is transmitted mainly through sex, injecting with shared needles, and from mother to child.

Sadly, many babies that escaped infection in the womb have become infected through breast-feeding.

Most women in African nations who are infected with HIV have been celibate before marriage but faithful since, but got infected by their husbands. Being female, poor and married can place someone at very high risk of infection.

Grief and pain for those left behind

Hundreds of millions of people have never heard of AIDS or are ignorant about how it spreads. In rural parts of India, most women don't know that sexual relationships can spread illnesses.

HIV does not kill directly, but it destroys the body's natural defences against disease. AIDS develops when the body succumbs to a secondary infection, often pneumonia or tuberculosis. Death may follow soon afterwards unless these infections are successfully treated.

There are many drugs which can prolong life but they have many side-effects and are still too expensive for most people with AIDS who live in the poorest nations. New programmes to provide low-cost or zero-cost treatment will not reach all areas, and the treatment requires medical tests every two weeks. Resistance to the medicine is common, and the pills have to be taken every day for life. Treatment of pregnant women makes it unlikely that their child will be infected at birth. There is no vaccine against HIV.

■ The above information is from Aids Care, Education and Training's website which can be found at www.acet-international.com

HIV prevention

Information from UNAIDS

Treatment and prevention challenge

- Expanding access to treatment is bringing hope to millions of people living with HIV – but this global movement must be matched with an equal commitment to expand access to HIV prevention services.
- Integrating prevention into treatment must be common practice – we must not sacrifice prevention at the expense of treatment. Today, less than one in five people worldwide has access to HIV prevention services and only 7% of people in developing countries have access to antiretrovirals.
- Only one out of nine people has access to voluntary counselling and testing. Stigma constitutes a major barrier to people coming forward for an HIV test. Knowledge of HIV status is the gateway to AIDS treatment and has documented prevention benefits.
- Expanding access to treatment is an incentive for people to get tested and know their status. It also reduces stigma, and can potentially bring millions into health-care settings to receive prevention interventions.
- Although HIV prevalence continues to rise in many countries, this should not be construed as a failure of proven prevention strategies, but rather a failure to ensure adequate access to these essential services.
- Without effective comprehensive prevention for all, the numbers of people living with HIV will continue to escalate, with disastrous short- and long-term effects.
- In high-income countries, prevention programmes must be reinvigorated to reduce prevailing prevention 'complacency' and to avoid the epidemic's resurgence.

Comprehensive prevention

- Comprehensive prevention involves all the strategies required to prevent transmission of HIV. These include AIDS education; behaviour change programmes for young people and other populations at higher risk of HIV exposure; promotion of male and female condoms, along with abstinence, being safer through fidelity and reducing the number of partners; voluntary counselling and testing; prevention of mother-to-child HIV transmission; preventing and treating sexually transmitted infections; blood safety, prevention of transmission in health-care settings; community education and changes in laws and policies to counter stigma; vulnerability reduction through social, legal and economic change; and harm reduction programmes for injecting drug users.
- Combination prevention refers to strategies to prevent sexual transmission of HIV. The 'A, B, Cs' of combination prevention are – Abstinence, Being safer (by being faithful or reducing the number of partners), and correct and consistent Condom use. A, B, and C interventions can be adapted and combined in a balanced approach that will vary depending on cultural context, the population targeted and the stage of the epidemic.
- For many women and girls in developing countries, the ABC approach is of limited value due to their lack of social and economic power. They cannot negotiate abstinence from sex, nor can they insist their partners remain faithful or use condoms.
- Effective prevention requires policies that help reduce the vulnerability of large numbers of people – in effect, creating a social, legal and economic environment in which prevention is possible. Initiatives that enhance economic and social development and

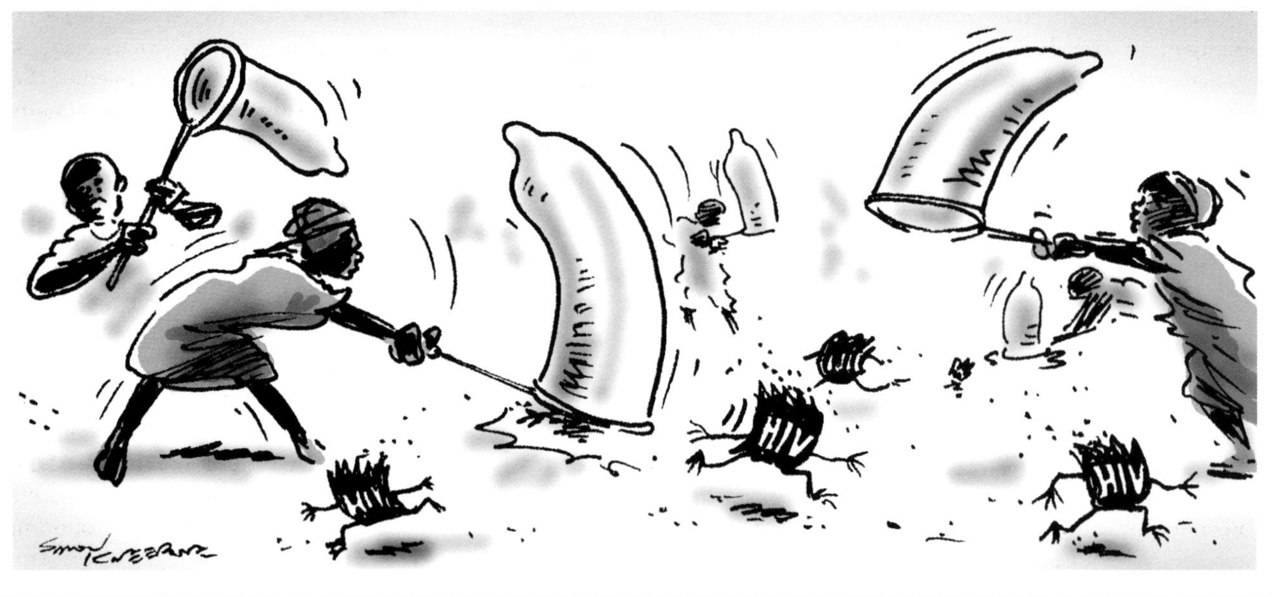

empower women and girls also contribute to effective AIDS responses.

Condoms and HIV prevention

- Condoms continue to be one of the most effective weapons in preventing the sexual transmission of HIV.
- Condoms have been found to be greater than 90% effective when used correctly and consistently.
- Evidence shows that condoms, when part of a broader prevention package, play a key role in reducing HIV infections and prevalence as seen in several countries, including Brazil, Cambodia, parts of Tanzania, Thailand, Uganda, and urban Zambia.
- More data are now emerging that demonstrate the effectiveness of condoms in preventing HIV transmission in generalized epidemics. A study from South Africa, soon to be published in the journal *AIDS*, finds that when enough young men use condoms consistently, there is a clear protective effect for both the individual and the population at large.

Condoms continue to be one of the most effective weapons in preventing the sexual transmission of HIV

- There is no evidence that promoting condoms leads to increased promiscuity among young people. Since the early 1990s, extensive research has shown that education about sexuality and access to condoms do not lead young people to begin having sex, or to have more partners.
- In fact, condoms, when distributed with educational materials as part of a combination prevention package, have been shown to delay sexual debut among those not sexually active. Among sexually active youth, HIV prevention education programmes have resulted in a reduced number of partners and increased condom use.
- The main reason that condoms can fail is due to improper use, breakage or slippage.
- Globally, condom distribution has increased substantially in recent years, but a large gap remains. According to UNFPA, the current supply of condoms is 40% short of what is needed. By 2015, an estimated 19 billion condoms will be needed to prevent HIV and other sexually transmitted infections. In Africa, despite progress made in some countries, current condom supplies fall far short – providing only three condoms per year for each adult male.
- While international funding for condoms peaked in 1996 at US$68 million, it subsequently declined to US$40 million annually in 1999 and 2000.

■ The above information is from UNAIDS' website: www.unaids.org

The future of HIV prevention

Information from the National AIDS Trust (NAT)

Current options for preventing HIV infection have not changed since the epidemic emerged in the 1980s: the same messages of abstinence, monogamy and condoms are the cornerstones of HIV prevention strategies. Yet HIV continues to be passed on because these methods do not address the factors that cause people to have sex.

These options are not realistic, and in some cases fail to protect people from many different walks of life: married couples, sex workers, women wanting to conceive and people living with HIV. There need to be more prevention options.

NAT campaigns for a much broader approach to HIV prevention not only to understand the full range of activity that needs to be in place to support and promote HIV prevention, but also to consider some of the new possibilities offered by HIV prevention technologies, such as vaccines and microbicides

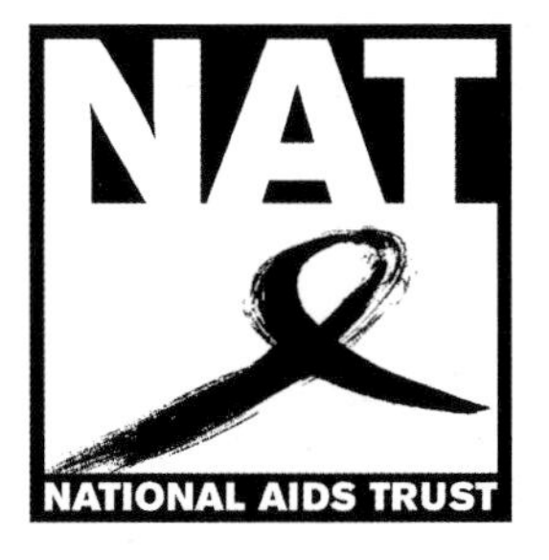

HIV vaccines and microbicides have the potential to make an enormous contribution towards ending the global HIV epidemic.

Vaccine

There is still no cure for AIDS. However, scientists have been working for many years to create a vaccine that would prevent HIV transmission in the same way many other infectious diseases (e.g. measles, smallpox and polio) are controlled. Such a vaccine is scientifically possible.

When will a vaccine be available?

There are 19 vaccines currently being tested in people around the world. It is hoped at least one vaccine would be available within ten years. However, the first generation of HIV vaccines are unlikely to be effective against the strains of HIV found in Africa and other parts of the developing world. A second generation of vaccines includes those designed for African strains of HIV, but is still in the early stages of development.

How much will it cost to produce a vaccine?

It has been estimated that it will cost US $1billion to create a safe, effective and affordable AIDS vaccine. Only US $430-470 million is currently invested worldwide on AIDS vaccine research and development. This is less than 1 per cent of spending on all health- and pharmaceutical-related research and development.

Who would be vaccinated?

HIV vaccines could not only be used to prevent infection occurring, but could also be given to people living with HIV as part of their treatment. In the UK, vaccines are likely to be provided to populations at high risk of HIV.

Does this mean the end of condoms?

No vaccine will be 100 per cent effective in preventing the spread of HIV. Vaccines will need to be integrated into existing prevention measures, including condom use, needle exchanges, education and behaviour change programmes. People will always need to reduce their risk of becoming infected regardless of whether a vaccine is available or not.

Microbicide

What is a microbicide?

A microbicide is a product, which used internally (vaginally or rectally) can prevent HIV transmission as well as offer protection against a variety of sexually transmitted infections (STIs). It could exist in the form of a gel, cream or suppository that could be active in the body for several hours. Microbicides are not to be confused with spermicides, which prevent contraception, although it is possible that a microbicide could also act as a contraceptive.

Are microbicides currently available?

No. There is currently no safe and effective microbicide available to the public. However, scientists are seriously pursuing over 60 product leads, including at least 12 that have proven safe and effective in animals and are now being tested in people. If one of these leads proves successful and investment is sufficient, a microbicide could be publicly available by 2008.

HIV vaccines could not only be used to prevent infection occurring, but could also be given to people living with HIV as part of their treatment

How would microbicides work?

Microbicides could work in several different ways. They could act as a liquid barrier to HIV entering the body, or strengthen the body's immune system to kill the virus. Alternatively, a microbicide could inactivate the virus before it is able to replicate within the blood stream. Microbicides would need to be applied before intercourse in order to be effective.

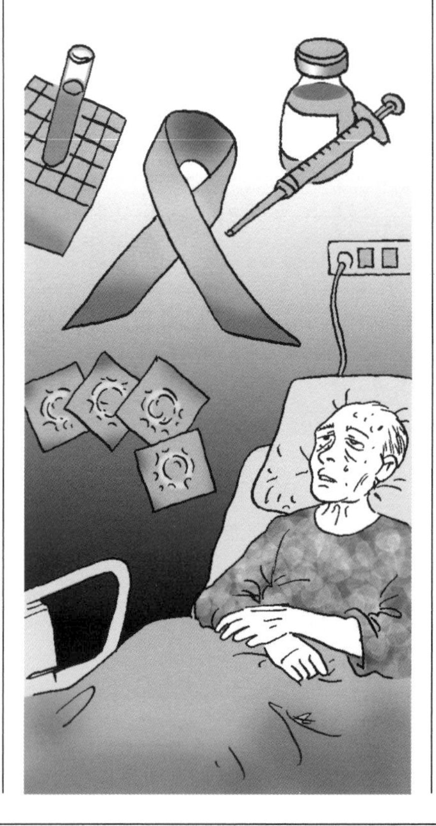

Who would use microbicides?

Many people could use a microbicide: gay or straight, married or single, HIV-positive or HIV-negative, old or young, male or female. Microbicides are not being developed in order to replace condoms, but to add to the options available for people who find consistent condom use hard to achieve.

In particular, global rates of new HIV infection among women, particularly young women, continue to rise disproportionately to infections in young men. In many developing countries, the greatest HIV risk factor for women is being married. It is vital that women and girls are empowered to protect themselves with a method they can directly control.

What is the future for HIV prevention?

NAT believes that new prevention technologies, including vaccines and microbicides, urgently need to be developed in order to broaden HIV prevention options. However, investment in this area must be complemented by renewed efforts to strengthen and expand education, condom distribution and behaviour change programmes.

In the UK, current HIV prevention efforts have numerous strengths, such as education for affected communities, a secure blood supply, a national programme of needle exchange and widespread access to anti-retroviral therapies. These have certainly contributed significantly to the UK's low levels of HIV transmission. However, the UK needs to begin to examine what new prevention technologies, such as a vaccine or a microbicide, might mean for the future of HIV education, individual gay men and Africans. It is also important to understand what impact these developments may have on sexual behaviour, how a partially effective vaccine and microbicide will be managed, and who will have access to vaccines and microbicides.

■ The above information is from National AIDS Trust's website which can be found at www.nat.org.uk

Treatment holds new promise in war on HIV

Microbicide gel could empower most at risk – married women

By Sarah Boseley in Bangkok

An HIV-killing gel called a microbicide – which women can apply long before intercourse and without a partner's knowledge – may be available in five to seven years, and is the best hope on the near horizon for checking the spread of HIV/Aids, researchers said 15 July 2004.

Microbicides can substantially reduce transmission of sexually transmitted infections when applied either in the vagina or rectum, and the cautious optimism over their development was a rare positive note on the last full day of the International Aids conference 15 July 2004.

The meeting in Bangkok has been dominated by disappointment at the slow progress in introducing drugs to save lives in poor countries while the numbers of those becoming infected and dying continue to soar.

Women in sub-Saharan Africa are increasingly being infected by the virus because they are often powerless to negotiate sex with their husbands. More married women are becoming infected than unmarried women, because their husbands are unfaithful and will not use condoms.

A weapon against HIV/Aids designed for women is urgently needed, Zeda Rosenberg, the chief executive of the International Partnership for Microbicides, told the conference 15 July 2004.

'Twenty-five per cent of women in South Africa are infected with HIV by the time they are 22 years old,' Dr Rosenberg said. 'In studies from Kenya and Zambia, adolescents who are married are contracting HIV at a faster rate than sexually active unmarried teenagers. And unfortunately parts of Asia are not far behind. So for women worldwide, being young and married are the most significant risk factors for acquiring HIV infection.'

She said the 'ABC' philosophy espoused by the United States government – abstinence, being faithful and using condoms – would not help. 'Married women, or women who do not have control over if they have sex, cannot choose abstinence. And many women who have contracted HIV infection from their husbands or long-term partners were faithful,' she said.

Four years ago at the Durban Aids conference, scientists revealed that trials of an early microbicide called nonoxynol-9, on which great hopes had been pinned, had been a catastrophic failure. It caused lesions in the cervix, which allowed the virus to enter the body.

But, Dr Rosenberg said, 'that was a detergent'. A number of other compounds are now in advanced trials which are not expected to cause damage. Talks have also been going on with the cosmetics industry to formulate compounds that do not cause irritation.

Dr Rosenberg predicted that a microbicide would be available in five to seven years. Even if it had limited efficacy – perhaps as low as 30% – it would save huge numbers of lives, she said. With vaccine research results disappointing, the microbicide looks likely to be the best bet for prevention in the near future.

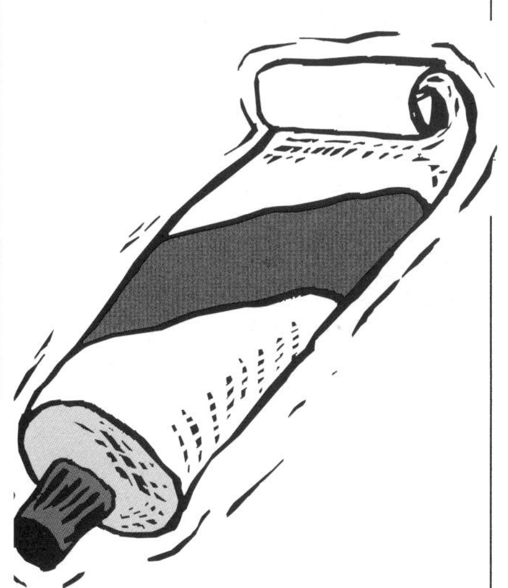

Britain has been at the forefront of the mission to develop a microbicide, which was backed with enthusiasm and cash by the former international development secretary Clare Short. The Medical Research Council in the UK has also been heavily involved.

Alan Stone, a virologist who chairs the UK-based International Working Group on Microbicides, said it was hoped that trials funded by the MRC and the Department for International Development of two polymer compounds would begin early next year. A trial of a surface-acting agent – like nonoxynol-9 but far milder – is already under way in Nigeria, and one involving a seaweed-based product is taking place in South Africa.

'Two to three years from now there will be a fairly clear indication of whether they are protective in these high-risk women,' he said.

Many candidates were needed to test the products, Dr Rosenberg told the conference. Her International Partnership is working on microbicides that could involve the antiretroviral drugs now used to treat people with HIV/Aids. Her organisation is involved in negotiations with the pharmaceutical companies that make the drugs.

There was much to do, she said, but 'failure is not an option'. She called for more money to be put into research.

'Unlike vaccines, there has been virtually no private sector investment in microbicide development,' she said.

Closing the treatment gap

Changing history

'3 by 5' is the global TARGET to get three million people living with HIV/AIDS in developing and middle-income countries on antiretroviral treatment by 2005.

It is a step towards the GOAL of providing universal access to treatment for all who need it as a human right.

Globally, between 35 and 42 million people are estimated to be infected with HIV/AIDS. Every single day AIDS kills 8,000 people and orphans thousands of children. Heavily affected countries face total social and economic collapse within just a few generations if decisive steps are not taken.

Antiretroviral therapy (ART) can keep people alive and transform HIV/AIDS from a death sentence to a manageable chronic disease. However, until now, treatment has been the most neglected area of HIV/AIDS programming.

The treatment gap facts

- Six million people need treatment now.
- Three million people die every year because they cannot get it.
- Worldwide only 440,000 people have access to treatment.
- In Africa, where 70% of people with HIV/AIDS live, ART is available to less than 4% of those in need.

At the United Nations General Assembly Special Session on HIV/AIDS in September 2003, the failure to deliver life-prolonging drugs to millions of people in need was declared a global health emergency. On World AIDS Day 2003 (December 1), the World Health Organization (WHO) and UNAIDS launched '3 by 5' – a global target to get three million people living with AIDS on antiretroviral treatment by the end of 2005. This target is a vital step towards the ultimate goal of providing universal access to AIDS treatment for all those who need it.

What will WHO do to contribute to '3 by 5'?

WHO provides support to developing countries in the form of simplified tools and guidelines and other forms of direct technical assistance for scaling up ART.

Globally, between 35 and 42 million people are estimated to be infected with HIV/AIDS. Every single day AIDS kills 8,000 people and orphans thousands of children

Procurement and management of pharmaceuticals and diagnostics pose a problem for most resource-limited countries. Therefore, WHO has established the AIDS Medicines and Diagnostics Service (AMDS) to assist countries with all aspects of selecting, procuring and delivering AIDS medicines and diagnostic tools to the point of service delivery.

To assist in reaching the '3 by 5' target, WHO and UNAIDS are focusing on key areas including:

- Providing simplified, standardised tools and treatment guidelines for ART in poor countries.
- Creating the new service (AMDS) to help countries to ensure an effective, reliable supply of medicines and diagnostics.
- Rapid identification, dissemination and application of new knowledge and successful strategies.
- Providing urgent, sustained support for countries to help with scale up of treatment.
- Providing assistance to countries and developing guidelines for capacity building and training

World must unite to meet the target

'3 by 5' is a global target that has been endorsed by 192 countries at

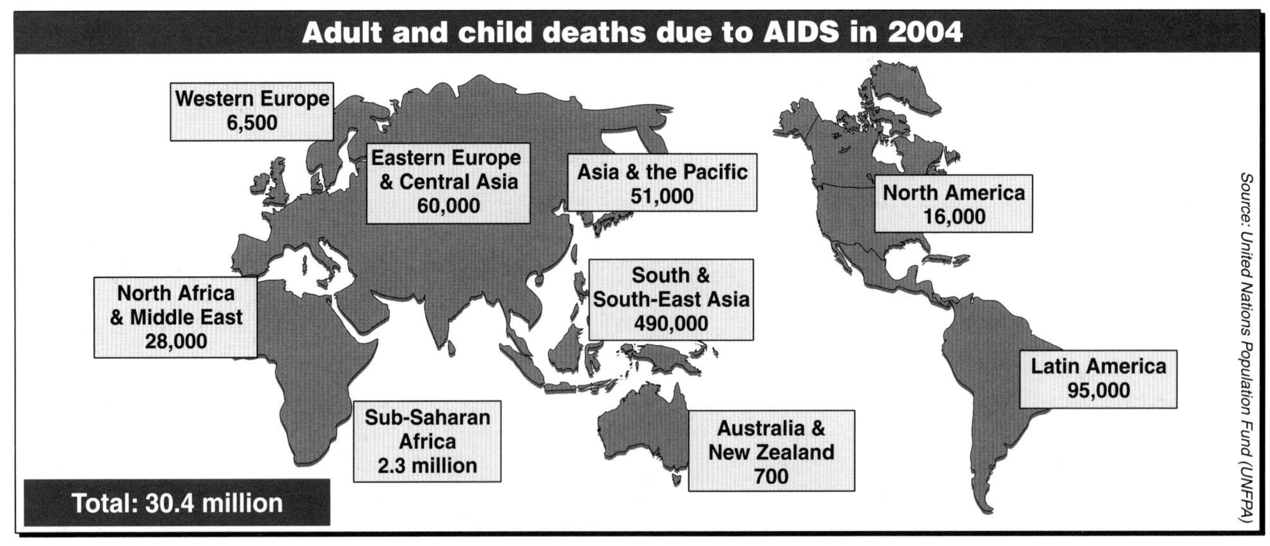

the World Health Assembly held in May 2004. Partnerships and collaboration at country and international level between national authorities, UN agencies, multilateral agencies, foundations, non-governmental, faith-based and community organisations, the private sector, labour unions and representatives of the community of people living with HIV/AIDS are absolutely essential if '3 by 5' is to be accomplished. Everybody has to play their part.

Why antiretroviral therapy (ART)?

ART prolongs lives, making HIV/AIDS a chronic disease, not a death sentence. Affluent countries have seen a 50 to 70% decline in HIV/AIDS deaths since the introduction of ART. ART will help reduce stigma and change attitudes towards HIV/AIDS. ART can significantly reduce HIV transmission. ART – once very costly – is now much more affordable in developing countries. ART can reduce overall health care costs and restore quality of life.

'Lack of access to antiretroviral therapy (ART) is a global health emergency. To deliver ART to the millions who need it, we must change the way we think and change the way we act.'

Dr Lee Jong-Wook, Director-General, World Health Organization

Treatment and prevention go together

To ensure a comprehensive response to HIV/AIDS, treatment and prevention programmes must enhance and accelerate each other. When people have hope that they can be treated and lead productive lives, the incentive to know their status and to protect themselves and their partners is much greater. Evidence and experience show that rapidly increasing the availability of ART leads to greater uptake of HIV testing. Availability of treatment, as well as enhanced community outreach, can lead to more openness about AIDS – which helps break down stigma and discrimination. People on effective treatment are also likely to be less infectious and less able to spread the virus.

Can it be done?

A growing number of countries have shown that increasing access to treatment is both possible and effective. Brazil has the most advanced national HIV/AIDS treatment programme in the developing world. It is estimated that between 1994 and 2002, almost 100,000 deaths have been averted in Brazil (a 50% drop in mortality) through the introduction of ART.

The programme in Brazil clearly demonstrates how scaling up can also help to strengthen health systems and dramatically reduce public health costs. As a result of the programme, there has been a significant decline in the number of hospital admissions. Cost savings in reduced hospital admissions and opportunistic infections are estimated at more than US $1 billion. The programme has also been effective in reducing the rates of TB and other opportunistic infections.

Making it easier

WHO has published guidelines to increase the availability of treatment in poor countries by recommending standardised treatment regimens and simplified approaches to clinical monitoring. These simplified guidelines also make it easier to train the thousands of health care workers needed to make scale up happen.

Fixed dose combinations

Fixed dose combinations (FDCs) of antiretroviral drugs are pills containing two or three AIDS drugs in one tablet. FDCs are a major breakthrough for AIDS treatment in poor countries as they offer significant operational advantages, including ease of distribution and storage, the likelihood of greater adherence, reduced incidence of treatment failure and drug resistance. Wherever possible, WHO recommends that FDCs be used in ART.

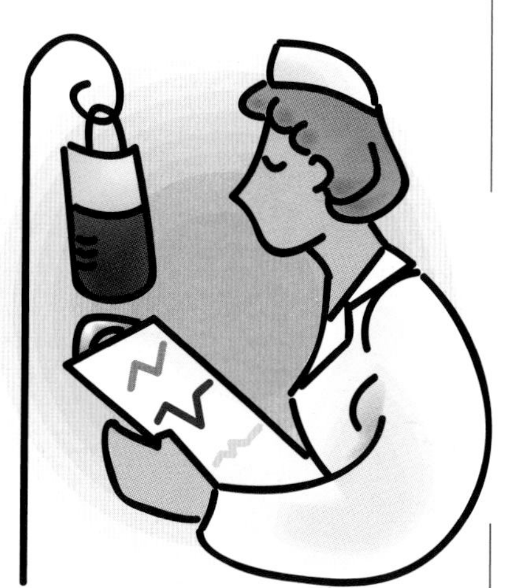

Prequalification

Countries most in need of life-saving antiretroviral and other drugs often do not have the regulatory capacity to ensure the safety and quality of medicines from different suppliers around the world. They often rely on procurement agencies, such as UNICEF and some non-governmental organisations, to purchase these medicines in bulk and distribute them. The Prequalification project, set up in 2001, is a service provided by WHO to facilitate the procurement of medicines that meet international standards of quality, safety and efficacy for HIV/AIDS, malaria and tuberculosis.

Prequalification was originally intended to give United Nations procurement agencies such as UNICEF the choice of a range of quality medicines. With time, the growing list of medicines that have been found to meet the set requirements has come to be seen as a useful tool for anyone purchasing medicines in bulk, including national governments and other organisations. For instance, the Global Fund to Fight AIDS, Tuberculosis and Malaria grants money for medicines that have been prequalified by the WHO process.

'This is a crucial moment in the history of HIV/AIDS, and an unprecedented opportunity to alter its course. The international community has the chance to change the history of health for generations to come and to open the door to better health for all.'

World Health Report 2004

■ The above information is from the World Health Organization. For further information visit their website at www.who.int

Responding to AIDS

Information from UNAIDS

AIDS is an extraordinary kind of crisis; it is both an emergency and a long-term development issue. Despite increased funding, political commitment and progress in expanding access to HIV treatment, the AIDS epidemic continues to outpace the global response. No region of the world has been spared. The epidemic remains extremely dynamic, growing and changing character as the virus exploits new opportunities for transmission.

Rates of infection are still on the rise in many countries in sub-Saharan Africa. In 2003 alone, an estimated 3 million people in the region became newly infected. New epidemics appear to be advancing unchecked in other places, notably Eastern Europe and Asia – regions that are experiencing the fastest-growing epidemics in the world.

More than 20 years and 20 million deaths since the first AIDS diagnosis in 1981, almost 38 million people (range 34. 6 -42. 3 million) are living with HIV. Even though the cure is elusive, we have learned crucial lessons about what works best in preventing new infections and improving the quality and care for people living with HIV. There have been some major developments, including antiretroviral medicines.

Despite these signs of progress, there are still huge challenges to turning the tide of this epidemic. Funding has greatly increased but is still only half of what is needed and is not always effectively utilised. Many national leaders remain in denial about the impact of AIDS on their people and societies.

Today we are faced with life and death choices. Without major action, the global epidemic will continue to outstrip the response. But there is an alternative: together we can forge policies grounded in science, not political rhetoric, and embark boldly on the 'Next Agenda' – an agenda for future action based on innovative approaches.

What are the major challenges?

- The female face of the epidemic. Women are increasingly at great risk of infection. As of December 2003, women accounted for nearly 50% of all people living with HIV worldwide and for 57% in sub-Saharan Africa. Women and girls also bear the brunt of the impact of the epidemic; they are most likely to take care of sick people, to lose jobs, income and schooling as a result of illness, and to face stigma and discrimination. There is an urgent need to address the many factors that contribute to women's vulnerability and risk – gender and cultural inequalities, violence, ignorance.
- Young people – 15- to 24-year-olds – account for nearly half of all new HIV infections worldwide. They are the largest youth generation in history and need a protective environment – regular schooling, access to health and support services – if they are to play their vital part in combating the epidemic.
- Scaling up treatment programmes providing life-prolonging anti-retroviral therapy. Only 7% of the people who need anti-retroviral treatment in developing countries have access to ARVs – 400,000 at the end of 2003. Programmes must be sustainable to prevent the development of drug-resistant strains of the virus.
- Several countries in southern Africa face a growing crisis in delivering vital public services that are crucial to the AIDS response. Reasons for this range from migration of key staff from public to private sectors, migration abroad, to the deadly impact of the AIDS epidemic itself.
- Scaling up prevention programmes that currently reach only one in five people at risk of HIV infection. In low- and middle-income countries in 2003, only one in ten pregnant women was offered services for preventing mother-to-child HIV transmission. In high-income countries, treatment has been a much higher priority than prevention and as a

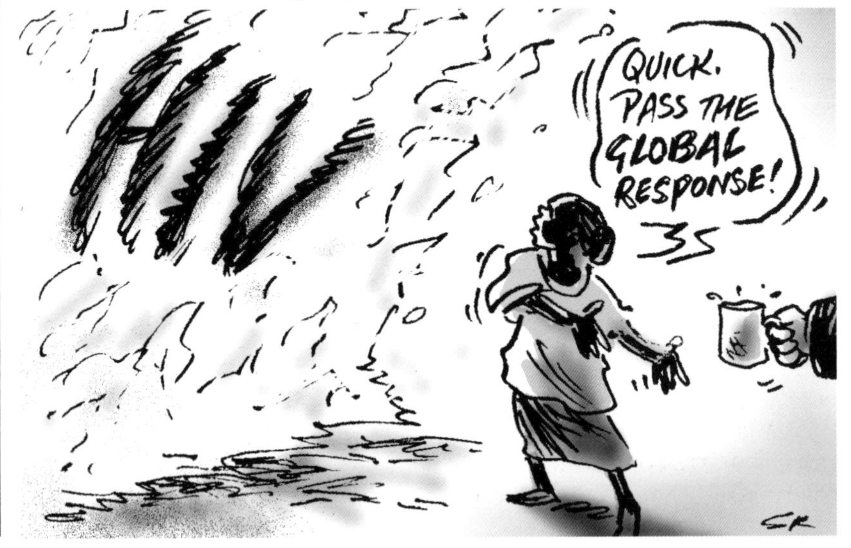

result, there have been rises in HIV transmission for the first time in a decade.

- Tackling stigma and discrimination. They directly hamper the effectiveness of AIDS responses stop people being tested for HIV, prevent the use of condoms or HIV-positive women breast-feeding to protect their babies against infection, and prevent marginalised groups such as injecting drug users receiving the care and support they need.
- Tackling the neglect of orphans. AIDS has killed one or both parents of an estimated 12 million children in sub-Saharan Africa and far too many of these orphans are not properly cared for.

Global AIDS funding

In addition to providing up-to-date global, regional and country data, the report releases new estimates on global resources needed to effectively combat the epidemic in the developing world. For the first time, the revised estimates reflect data obtained from 78 countries, many on the frontlines of the AIDS epidemic.

Although global spending on AIDS has increased 15-fold from US$300 million in 1996 to just under US$5 billion in 2003, it is less than half of what will be needed by 2005 in developing countries. According to newly revised costing estimates, an estimated US$12 billion (up from US$10 billion) will be needed by 2005 and US$20 billion by 2007 for prevention and care in low- and middle-income countries.

The estimated US$20 billion would provide antiretroviral therapy to just over six million people (over four million in sub-Saharan Africa), support for 22 million orphans, HIV voluntary counselling and testing for 100 million adults, school-based AIDS education for 900 million students and peer counselling services for 60 million young people not in school. About 43% of these resources will be needed in sub-Saharan Africa, 28% in Asia, 17% in Latin American and the Caribbean, 9% in Eastern Europe, and 1% in North Africa and the Near East.

Fully funding the response to AIDS will require an extraordinary effort, which cannot be met from currently planned regular domestic and international development budgets. It will require extraordinary leadership and will have to use currently untapped resources.

■ The above information is an extract from the *2004 Report on the global AIDS epidemic: Executive Summary*, produced by UNAIDS. For further information visit their website at www.unaids.org

Government 'letting up on Aids battle'

By James Meikle, Health Correspondent

The government was accused 8 August 2004 of failing to tackle the HIV/Aids crisis in its own back yard while focusing on trying to help the international battle against the disease.

The National Aids Trust said sexual health had dropped off the list of national priorities with anti-HIV funds no longer ring-fenced. This has meant a drop in education and prevention programmes and long waiting times for tests.

People at high risk of infection, including prostitutes and injecting drug users, were treated as criminals while the NHS's attitude towards failed asylum seekers needed reviewing.

The trust said political leadership, cross-government co-ordination and a respect for human rights were all lacking. It said Britain had failed to honour a commitment made in 2001 to report to the UN on targets regarding HIV issues.

There were an estimated 7,000 new cases of HIV infection in Britain last year, taking the total to about 50,000, a third of them undiagnosed. There have been increases in heterosexual transmission, particularly within the African community.

In July 2004, doctors at sexual health clinics said the Home Office policy of dispersing asylum seekers risked spreading the disease because it could interrupt therapy and compromise care.

There were an estimated 7,000 new cases of HIV infection in Britain last year, taking the total to about 50,000, a third of them undiagnosed

But there is also mounting unease over planned guidance for GPs that will state that failed asylum seekers will only have free access to free emergency or 'immediately necessary' treatment.

That means they would have to pay for other treatments, such as anti-retroviral drugs, when they are banned from working or receiving benefits.

Similar rules limiting access to free treatment for those who have been refused permission to stay in Britain have been introduced for hospitals.

Campaigners are furious that the package to prevent 'health tourism' takes in failed asylum seekers because it could hinder attempts to tackle HIV.

KEY FACTS

■ Since 1995, there has been a sustained increase in diagnoses of most STIs (also called STDs) in the UK. (p. 2)

■ There are 1.5 million attendances at genitourinary medicine clinics in the UK each year, a number which has been growing by at least 15% annually. (p. 3)

■ The number of new cases of syphilis showed the highest increase between 2002 and 2003 with a rise of 28%, while diagnoses of chlamydia went up by 9% in the same period. (p. 4)

■ Sexually transmitted infections don't always cause symptoms, so a checkup and tests are often needed to tell if you have an infection. (p. 10)

■ 'Fast access to treatment is essential to prevent the spread of infection and makes economic sense, yet waiting times are as long as six weeks.' (p. 11)

■ HIV is short for Human Immunodeficiency Virus. HIV attacks the body's immune system, making it hard to fight off infections. (p. 14)

■ AIDS stands for Acquired Immune Deficiency Syndrome. When a person's immune system has been damaged he or she is open to other illnesses, especially infections (e.g. tuberculosis and pneumonia) and cancers, many of which would not normally be a threat. (p. 14)

■ The number of new cases of HIV diagnosed in the UK has risen by 20% in one year, according to figures released by the Health Protection Agency. There have been 5,047 new cases so far for 2003, compared with 4,204 at the same time last year. (p. 16)

■ The overwhelming majority of people with HIV – some 95 per cent of the global total – live in the developing world. (p. 17)

■ Half of new infections are occurring in young people (15- to 24-year-olds), who constitute over one-quarter of those living with HIV and AIDS worldwide. (p. 17)

■ In western Europe, deaths from AIDS have declined due to the availability of HIV treatment. Alarmingly, AIDS infection rates have continued to rise because of waning government commitments to prevention efforts and complacency linked to the availability of treatment. (p. 19)

■ Prevention is key to halting the growing AIDS epidemic. People need to be educated about the possible impact of risky behaviour and have access to condoms, needle exchange programmes and substitution therapy. (p. 19)

■ According to the National Association of NHS Providers of AIDS Care and Treatment (PACT), the cost of managing a patient with HIV is £15,000 per year. The total cost of treatment and care in 2002-03 will be £345 million. (p. 21)

■ Biologically, the risk of infection during unprotected sex is two to four times higher for women than men; young women are even more vulnerable because their reproductive tracts are still maturing and tears in the tissue allow easy access to infection. (p. 24)

■ Because sex is a taboo topic in many countries, large numbers of young people do not get sufficient information – or the skills – to refuse sex or negotiate safer sex practices. (p. 25)

■ HIV/AIDS has become a disease of young people, with half of all new infections occurring in 15- to 24-year-olds, according to UNFPA's *The State of World Population 2003* report. (p. 29)

■ The fastest spread of HIV/AIDS among youth is in sub-Saharan Africa, where an estimated 8.6 million youth (67 per cent female) are infected, followed by South Asia where some 1.1 million youth are infected (62 per cent female). (p. 29)

■ 'Sexual and reproductive health and Aids are inextricably linked. By taking action on one, we know we are also helping to tackle the other.' (p. 31)

■ HIV does not kill directly, but it destroys the body's natural defences against disease. AIDS develops when the body succumbs to a secondary infection, often pneumonia or tuberculosis. Death may follow soon afterwards unless these infections are successfully treated. (p. 31)

■ Expanding access to treatment is bringing hope to millions of people living with HIV – but this global movement must be matched with an equal commitment to expand access to HIV prevention services. (p. 32)

■ There is still no cure for AIDS. However, scientists have been working for many years to create a vaccine that would prevent HIV transmission in the same way many other infectious diseases (e.g. measles, smallpox and polio) are controlled. Such a vaccine is scientifically possible. (p. 33)

■ Britain has been at the forefront of the mission to develop a microbicide, which was backed with enthusiasm and cash by the former international development secretary Clare Short. The Medical Research Council in the UK has also been heavily involved. (p. 35)

■ Globally, between 35 and 42 million people are estimated to be infected with HIV/AIDS. Every single day AIDS kills 8,000 people and orphans thousands of children. (p. 36)

■ Although global spending on AIDS has increased 15-fold from US$300 million in 1996 to just under US$5 billion in 2003, it is less than half of what will be needed by 2005 in developing countries. (p. 39)

ADDITIONAL RESOURCES

You might like to contact the following organisations for further information. Due to the increasing cost of postage, many organisations cannot respond to enquiries unless they receive a stamped, addressed envelope.

Aids Care, Education and Training (ACET)
1 Carlton Gardens
Ealing
London, W5 2AN
Tel: 020 8567 9824
E-mail: acet@acetuk.org
Website: www.acet-international.com
ACET International Alliance is a rapidly growing global network of independent Christian organisations and church-based agencies responding to AIDS, run and staffed almost in every case by nationals. We are united in a race against time to prevent another generation in African nations and elsewhere being devastated by AIDS, and to provide help to the sick, dying and bereaved.

AVERT
4 Brighton Road
Horsham
West Sussex, RH13 5BA
Tel: 01403 210202
Fax: 01403 211001
E-mail: info@avert.org
Website: www.avert.org
AVERT is a leading UK AIDS Education and Medical Research charity. They are responsible for a wide range of education and medical research work. They produce a wide range of free resources on their website.

Brook
Unit 421, Highgate Studios
53-79 Highgate Road
London, NW5 1TL
Tel: 020 7284 6040
Fax: 020 7284 6050
E-mail: admin@brookcentres.org.uk
Website: www.brook.org.uk
Brook is the only national voluntary sector provider of free and confidential sexual health advice and services specifically for young people under 25. Young people can call Brook free and in confidence on 0800 0185 023 or by online enquiry via Ask Brook at www.brook.org.uk

fpa (formerly The Family Planning Association)
2-12 Pentonville Road
London, N1 9FP
Tel: 020 7837 5432
Fax: 020 7837 3042
Website: www.fpa.org.uk
Produces information and publications on all aspects of reproduction and sexual health – phone for a publications catalogue. The Helpline on 020 7837 4044 Monday-Friday 9am to 7pm is run by qualified healthcare workers and can answer queries on all aspects of family planning.

NAM Publications
16a Clapham Common South Side
London, SW4 7AB
Tel: 020 7627 3200
Website: www.aidsmap.com
NAM is an award-winning, community-based organisation, which works from the UK. Delivers reliable and accurate HIV information across the world to HIV-positive people and to the professionals who treat, support and care for them.

National AIDS Trust (NAT)
New City Cloisters
196 Old Street
London, EC1V 9FR
Tel: 020 7814 6767
Fax: 020 7216 0111
E-mail: info@nat.org.uk
Website: www.nat.org.uk
The National AIDS Trust aims to promote a wider understanding of HIV and AIDS, develop and support efforts to prevent the spread of HIV, and improve the quality of life of people affected by HIV and AIDS.

Terrence Higgins Trust
52-54 Gray's Inn Road
London, WC1X 8JU
Tel: 020 7831 0330
Fax: 020 7242 0121
E-mail: info@tht.org.uk
Website: www.tht.org.uk
THT is the leading HIV & AIDS charity in the UK and the largest in Europe. It was one of the first charities to be set up in response to the HIV epidemic and has been at the forefront of the fight against HIV & AIDS ever since.

UK Coalition of People Living with HIV and AIDS
250 Kennington Lane
London
SE11 5RD
Tel: 020 7564 2121
Fax: 020 7564 2128
E-mail: editor@positivenation.co.uk
Website: www.ukcoalition.org
www.positivenation.co.uk
Positive Nation is the UK's HIV and sexual health magazine.

United Nations Population Fund (UNFPA)
220 East 42nd Street
New York NY10017
USA
Tel: + 1 212 297 5279
Fax: + 1 212 557 6416
E-mail: hq@unfpa.org
Website: www.unfpa.org
UNFPA, the United Nations Population Fund, helps developing countries find solutions to their population problems. Publishes *The State of World Population*, an annual report highlighting new developments in population. Also publishes many other titles and information on various aspects of the issue of population.

World Health Organization (WHO)
Avenue Appia 20
1211 Geneva 27
Switzerland
Tel: + 41 22 791 2111
Fax: + 41 22 791 3111
E-mail: info@who.int
Website: www.who.int
WHO works to make a difference in the lives of the world's people by enhancing both life expectancy and health expectancy.

INDEX

ACKNOWLEDGEMENTS

The publisher is grateful for permission to reproduce the following material.

While every care has been taken to trace and acknowledge copyright, the publisher tenders its apology for any accidental infringement or where copyright has proved untraceable. The publisher would be pleased to come to a suitable arrangement in any such case with the rightful owner.

Chapter One: Sexual Health

Sexually transmitted infections, © Brook, *Sexually transmitted diseases in the UK*, © AVERT, *United Kingdom STD statistics*, © AVERT, *Sex infections rise again*, © Guardian Newspapers Limited 2004, *Selected conditions by sex*, © Crown copyright is reproduced with the permission of Her Majesty's Stationery Office, *Sexually transmitted infections*, © fpa, *Young, free and infectious*, © Guardian Newspapers Limited 2004, *Sexual health check-ups*, © NAM Publications 2004, *Patients wait six weeks to visit sex disease clinics*, © Guardian Newspapers Limited 2004, *Unprotected sex*, © NAM Publications 2004, *Exposure category of HIV infection*, © Crown copyright is reproduced with the permission of Her Majesty's Stationery Office, *Men and sexual health*, © Brook.

Chapter Two: HIV & AIDS

HIV facts, © Terrence Higgins Trust, *New HIV cases up by a fifth in a year*, © Guardian Newspapers Limited 2004, *Global statistics*, © National AIDS Trust, *HIV and AIDS around the world*, © National AIDS Trust, *AIDS epidemic poses serious threat to Europe*, © World Health Organization 2004, *HIV/AIDS FAQs*, © AVERT, *New warning over the fast-growing HIV threat*, © Guardian Newspapers Limited 2004, *HIV/AIDS and adolescents*, © United Nations Population Fund (UNFPA), *Young people and HIV/AIDS*, © UNICEF/UNAIDS/WHO, *New HIV infections in 2002*, © UNAIDS, *Carry on up the campus*, © UK Coalition of People Living with HIV and AIDS, *HIV/AIDS now a disease of young people . . .*, © United Nations Population Fund (UNFPA), *Adults and children living with HIV/AIDS*, © United Nations Population Fund (UNFPA), *Record numbers infected*, © Guardian Newspapers Limited 2004, *AIDS pandemic out of control in many nations*, © Aids Care, Education and Training (ACET), *HIV prevention*, © UNAIDS, *The future of HIV prevention*, © National AIDS Trust, *Treatment holds new promise in war on HIV*, © Guardian Newspapers Limited 2004, *Closing the treatment gap*, © World Health Organization 2004, *Adult and child deaths due to AIDS in 2004*, © United Nations Population Fund (UNFPA), *Responding to AIDS*, © UNAIDS, *Government 'letting up on Aids battle'*, © Guardian Newspapers Limited 2004.

Photographs and illustrations:

Pages 1, 16, 23, 32, 38: Simon Kneebone; pages 2, 14, 34: Angelo Madrid; page 7, 21: Pumpkin House; pages 8, 19, 27: Don Hatcher; pages 11, 30: Bev Aisbett.

Craig Donnellan
Cambridge
January, 2005